TWO PATHS DIVERGED

The Highs, Lows, And Hows of Hiking

BY BRIAN C EBY

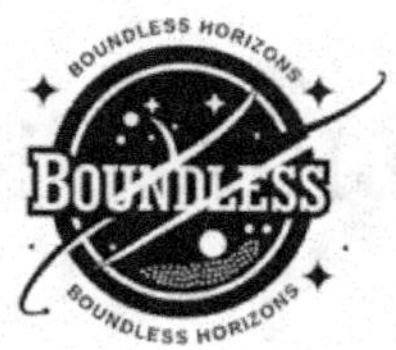

TABLE OF CONTENTS

PREFACE ix

CHAPTER 1: THE HISTORY OF HIKING 1

Introduction 1

The Early Days of Hiking...1

The Genesis of Hiking...2

Pilgrimages: The Spiritual Journeys 2

Exploration and Discovery 4

The Influence of the Romantic Movement 4

Transition to Leisure 5

CHAPTER 2: TYPES OF HIKING AND THE BENEFITS 7

Understanding Hiking - Definitions and Types...7

Defining Hiking 7

Types of Hiking 8

The Physical and Mental Benefits 11

Physical Health Benefits 12

Mental Health Benefits 13

Long-Term Mental Health Benefits 15

Understanding Hiking - Hiking as a Form of Eco-Tourism 16

Hiking and Eco-Tourism: A Natural Synergy......................................16

The Benefits of Hiking for Eco-Tourism...16

Challenges of Hiking as Eco-Tourism...18

Best Practices for Hiking as Eco-Tourism 18

CHAPTER 3 PREPARING FOR THE HIKE - PHYSICAL PREPARATION AND

CONDITIONING 21

Understanding the Demands of Hiking...21

Building Endurance 22

Strengthening Muscles..23

Enhancing Balance and Flexibility 23

Practical Training: Simulating Hiking Conditions............................24

Listening to Your Body and Rest 25

Nutrition and Hydration..25

Preparing for the Hike - Essential Gear and How to Select It................26

Footwear: The Foundation of Every Hike..26

Backpacks: Carrying Your Essentials 26
Clothing: Dressing for Success 27
Navigation Tools: Staying on Course...27
First Aid Kit: Preparedness for Emergencies 28
Hydration Systems: Staying Hydrated..28
Nutrition: Fueling Your Body..28
Lighting: Illuminating Your Path 29
Shelter: Protection from the Elements 29
Multi-Tool and Repair Kits: Readiness for Repairs 30
Understanding Your Nutritional Needs..31
Carbohydrates...31
Proteins 31
Fats..32
Planning Your Meals and Snacks...32
Hydration Strategies 33
Tips for Eating and Drinking on the Trail......................................34
Pre-Hike and Post-Hike Nutrition 35
Special Considerations..35
Necessary Skills 36
The Basics of Map Reading 36
Compass Skills 37
GPS and Electronic Navigation 38
Navigating Without a Compass or GPS 39
Practical Navigation Tips 39
Advanced Navigation Techniques..40
Conclusion...41
Environmental Hazards...42
Wildlife Encounters..43
Getting Lost..44
Personal Safety Measures...44
Group Dynamics...46
Essential First Aid 47
Assessing the Situation 47
Common Injuries and Conditions..47
When to Seek Further Medical Help 49

Wilderness First Aid Courses 50

Trail Etiquette 50

Right-of-Way on the Trail 51

Minimizing Environmental Impact 51

Respectful Interactions 52

Camping Etiquette 53

Managing Conflicts 54

Implementation in Hiking 58

Making the Choice 110

The Future of Navigation and Tracking Technologies 118

Understanding the Landscape 119

The Science of Light 120

Ethical Considerations and Conservation 122

GEAR LIST TEMPLATES 163

Trip Planner Template 1...163

Trip Planner Template 2...165

GLOSSARY 168

The Road Less Traveled
- Robert Frost

Two roads diverged in a yellow wood,
And sorry I could not travel both
And be one traveler, long I stood
And looked down one as far as I could
To where it bent in the undergrowth;

Then took the other, as just as fair,
And having perhaps the better claim,
Because it was grassy and wanted wear;
Though as for that the passing there
Had worn them really about the same,

And both that morning equally lay
In leaves no step had trodden black.
Oh, I kept the first for another day!
Yet knowing how way leads on to way,
I doubted if I should ever come back.

I shall be telling this with a sigh
Somewhere ages and ages hence:
Two roads diverged in a wood, and I—
I took the one less traveled by,
And that has made all the difference.

PREFACE

Welcome to "Two Paths Diverged: The Highs, Lows, And Hows Of Hiking," a book that endeavors to be your companion, guide, and inspiration on all trails, whether you're setting foot on a path for the first time or are a seasoned hiker with countless miles under your belt. This book is the culmination of years spent traversing diverse landscapes, from the bamboo forests of ancient lands to the rugged Rocky peaks that pierce the sky. Through these pages, I aim to share the knowledge and practical advice accumulated over these journeys and sometimes the challenges hiking presents.

This book is written to inspire you to explore the natural world, armed with respect for its beauty and an understanding of how to tread lightly upon it. Whether your interest lies in short day hikes to escape city life, ambitious backpacking trips through remote wilderness, or the pursuit of conquering the trails that stretch across continents, there is something in these pages for you.

"Two Paths Diverged" is structured to guide you through every aspect of hiking. It starts by looking back at the history of hiking, tracing the evolution of this pastime from a necessary mode of travel to a popular leisure activity and a form of eco-tourism. Understanding the roots of hiking enriches our appreciation of the trail and highlights the importance of preserving these natural spaces for future generations.

As we delve into the practical aspects of hiking, you'll find chapters on preparing for your hike, from physical conditioning and selecting the right gear to mastering navigation and ensuring your safety in the wilderness. Respecting nature and practicing Leave No Trace principles are emphasized, promoting an ethical approach to outdoor adventures.

Advanced hiking techniques and technology integration into our hiking experiences are covered, reflecting the modern hiker's toolkit. The discussion extends to the digital realm, examining how social media and mobile applications have transformed how we hike, share, and preserve our adventures.

In closing, "Two Paths Diverged: The Highs, Lows, And Hows Of Hiking" is more than just a guidebook. It is an invitation to embark on a journey of challenge and fulfillment. Hiking offers a unique blend of physical exertion, mental relaxation, and rejuvenation. It teaches us resilience, humility, and the sheer joy of reaching a summit or completing a challenging trek. This book aims to share these benefits with you and may it catalyze your adventures and be a reminder of the incredible beauty our planet offers to those willing to explore it on foot.

The journey through the hiking world is as varied and diverse as the landscapes we traverse. Each step is a step toward learning about the environment that sustains us. My sincerest wish is that you will find a path to personal discovery and an honest connection to the planet through hiking.

ONE

THE HISTORY OF HIKING

Introduction

Hiking, a word that evokes images of lush forests, towering peaks, and trails leading into the unknown, has a history as rich and varied as the landscapes it traverses. Today's activity draws millions of enthusiasts worldwide, each seeking something unique on their journey—be it adventure, solitude, or a deeper connection with nature. But to truly grasp the essence of hiking, we must first delve into its origins, tracing the evolution from necessity to leisure, and recognize the milestones that have shaped it into the modern pursuit we know today.

The Early Days of Hiking

The history of hiking, as we understand it today—a recreational pursuit infused with a sense of adventure, exploration, and appreciation for nature—is deeply rooted in the early days of human civilization.

The Genesis of Hiking

Walking was a fundamental aspect of human life, essential for hunting, gathering, and migrating across ancient Earth's vast, untamed landscapes. These early humans, our ancestors, developed an intimate knowledge of the land, following animal trails, rivers, and mountain passes, learning the rhythms of nature. This profound connection with the environment was not hiking for leisure but a symbiotic relationship with the earth, critical for survival, and it is this deep respect and appreciation for nature that we aim to instill in every hiker.

As civilizations grew, so did the complexity of human interaction with the land. Ancient trade routes, like the Silk Road connecting the East and West, were traversed by traders and pilgrims, expanding cultural exchanges and commerce. These journeys, though primarily for trade, required an extensive understanding of navigation, endurance, and the natural world, laying the groundwork for the development of hiking. This historical significance and global impact of hiking is something we should all be aware of as we embark on our own hiking journeys.

Pilgrimages: The Spiritual Journeys

A significant transformation in walking came with the rise of religious pilgrimages. These spiritual quests, undertaken for penance, enlightenment, or devotion, became a form of early hiking, engaging people with the physical and mental challenges of long-distance walking.

- **The Camino de Santiago:** Perhaps the most renowned pilgrimage of the medieval era, the Camino de Santiago drew (and continues to draw) thousands of pilgrims annually. Originating in various locations across Europe, the routes converge in Santiago de Compostela, Spain, where the shrine of Saint James the Apostle is located. With its network of routes, this pilgrimage promoted walking as a spiritual endeavor. It contributed to developing the infrastructure, such as hostels and marked trails, that would later support recreational hiking.

- **The Via Francigena:** Another notable pilgrimage is the Via Francigena, a route stretching from Canterbury, England, to Rome, Italy. Pilgrims in the medieval period walked this route seeking the holy city of Rome, navigating through diverse terrains across several countries. Like the Camino de Santiago, the Via Francigena fostered an early culture of long-distance walking, uniting people with a common goal.

These pilgrimages were among the first instances where walking transcended its utility, becoming imbued with meaning, community, and a sense of achievement. They laid the foundational ethos of hiking: endurance, exploration, and the pursuit of a goal.

Exploration and Discovery

Starting in the 15th century, the Age of Exploration introduced a new dimension to walking exploration. Explorers, driven by the desire for new knowledge, wealth, and territories, ventured into the unknown, mapping the world one step at a time. These expeditions required incredible feats of endurance and navigation, pushing the boundaries of human understanding of the globe.

- **Lewis and Clark Expedition:** One of the most famous exploration hikes in American history, the Lewis and Clark Expedition (1804-1806), commissioned by President Thomas Jefferson, sought a route to the Pacific Ocean. This journey of over 8,000 miles on foot, by boat, and on horseback through uncharted American territories highlighted the critical role of walking in exploration. The expedition's success in mapping the West and documenting its natural resources, landscapes, and inhabitants underscored walking as a tool for discovery.

The Influence of the Romantic Movement

The Romantic Movement of the late 18th and early 19th centuries marked a turning point in the perception of nature. This cultural movement, emphasizing emotion, individualism, and the sublime beauty of the natural world, inspired a newfound appreciation for landscapes and the outdoors.

- **The Lake District:** In England, the Lake District became a focal point for the Romantics, captivated by its dramatic natural scenery. Avid walkers and poets like William Wordsworth and Samuel Taylor Coleridge celebrated the spiritual and aesthetic pleasure of walking in nature. In his guide to the Lakes, Wordsworth described walking as a divine act, enriching the soul and mind. This sentiment resonated with many, elevating walking in nature from a mundane activity to a revered, almost sacred, pursuit.

Transition to Leisure

As the 19th century progressed, the foundations laid by pilgrimages, exploration, and the Romantic Movement converged, setting the stage for hiking as a recreational activity. The Industrial Revolution, while urbanizing societies, also engendered a longing for the natural world, now seen as an escape from the smoke and noise of cities. This yearning, combined with the Romantic idealization of nature, made walking in the countryside increasingly popular among the burgeoning middle class, eager for leisure activities that provided physical health benefits and mental solace.

- **The Birth of Recreational Hiking:** This era saw the emergence of the first hiking clubs and organizations dedicated to enjoying and preserving the natural world. In Britain, the Sunday Tramps, a group of enthusiasts led by poet Leslie Stephen (father of Virginia Woolf), began organizing regular walks in the countryside, embodying the spirit of recreational hiking. Similarly, in the United States, the Appalachian Mountain Club, founded in 1876 and later the Sierra Club in 1892, marked the formalization of hiking as a leisure activity, emphasizing the enjoyment of nature and its conservation.

The early days of hiking, from the primal necessity of walking through spiritual pilgrimages and exploring new lands to the Romantic Movement's celebration of nature, have collectively shaped hiking into a multifaceted activity. It became a pursuit that offered physical challenge and exploration, spiritual fulfillment, and a profound connection with the natural world. This rich tapestry of influences set the stage for the modern hiking movement, a testament to the enduring human desire to walk, explore, and connect with the earth.

TWO

TYPES OF HIKING
AND THE BENEFITS

Understanding Hiking - Definitions and Types

Hiking, a term that evokes wide-ranging images from serene walks in the woods to challenging treks up steep mountain passes, encompasses a variety of experiences defined by the terrain, distance, and purpose of the walk. As a form of recreation, exercise, and, at times, a spiritual journey, hiking appeals to a diverse group of people worldwide. This chapter explores the multifaceted nature of hiking, clarifying its definitions and delving into the various types that have evolved to cater to different preferences and skill levels.

Defining Hiking

At its core, hiking is going for long, vigorous walks, typically on trails or footpaths in the countryside. It's a simple yet profound activity that connects humans with nature, offering physical challenges, mental relaxation, and a sense of adventure. Unlike other forms of travel, hiking emphasizes the journey rather than the destination, encouraging a slow, deliberate exploration of the natural world.

The definition of hiking, however, can vary significantly depending on cultural context and personal interpretation. For some, a hike is a multi-day trek through remote wilderness, requiring extensive preparation and survival skills. For others, it's a leisurely day walk in a local park. This broad definition speaks to the inclusivity of hiking as an activity accessible to people of all ages, fitness levels, and backgrounds.

Types of Hiking

To better understand the spectrum of hiking experiences, it's helpful to categorize them into distinct types. These classifications help potential hikers identify what kind of adventure they're seeking and what they need to prepare for it.

- **Day Hiking:** Day hikes are the most accessible form of hiking, suitable for people of all ages and fitness levels. These hikes typically last several hours and do not require overnight camping. Trails range from easy walks on well-maintained paths to challenging routes involving significant elevation changes or rugged terrain. Day hiking is an excellent way to enjoy the outdoors without the commitment of a more extended expedition.

- **Backpacking:** Backpacking extends the hiking experience over multiple days and involves camping in the wilderness or designated campsites. This type of hiking requires carrying all necessary gear and provisions in a backpack, including food, water, shelter, and clothing. Backpacking trails can vary widely in difficulty and terrain, offering adventurers a deeper immersion into nature and the challenge of self-sufficiency.

- **Thru-hiking** refers to completing a long-distance trail, often stretching hundreds or thousands of miles. Famous examples include the Appalachian Trail, the Pacific Crest Trail, and the Continental Divide Trail in the United States. Thru-hiking is a demanding endeavor that requires months of planning, preparation, and physical and mental resilience. It's a transformative experience that many hikers find deeply rewarding.

- **Section Hiking:** Section hiking is a method of completing a long-distance trail by hiking individual sections over time rather than in a single continuous journey. This approach allows hikers to tackle challenging trails at their own pace, making long-distance hiking more accessible to those with limited time or resources.

- **Ultralight Hiking:** Ultralight hiking is a minimalist approach to backpacking, where hikers aim to carry the lightest and simplest gear possible. The goal is to reduce pack weight to a minimum, often to less than 10 pounds (excluding food and water), to increase mobility and enjoy a more comfortable hiking experience. Ultralight hiking requires careful gear selection and a willingness to forego certain comforts.

- **Peak Bagging:** Peak bagging is the practice of hiking to the summits of mountains. It often involves a checklist of peaks to "bag," ranging from local high points to famous mountains like the Seven Summits—the highest peak on each continent. Peak baggers seek the physical challenge and sense of accomplishment of reaching a summit.

- **Adventure Hiking:** Adventure hiking incorporates elements of other outdoor activities, such as rock climbing, rappelling, or river crossing, into the hiking experience. These hikes are typically more technical and require specialized skills and equipment. Adventure hiking offers an adrenaline-fueled variation for those looking for more than a traditional trail walk.

- **Social Hiking:** Social hiking emphasizes the communal aspect of hiking, focusing on enjoying nature in the company of others. Hiking clubs, group outings, and organized events fall under this category, providing opportunities for social interaction, shared experiences, and the formation of friendships based on a love of the outdoors.

- **Solo Hiking:** Unlike social hiking, solo hiking involves hiking alone, offering solitude, reflection, and a personal connection with nature. Solo hikers can move at their own pace, make decisions, and experience the wilderness on their own terms. While solo hiking can be deeply rewarding, it also requires careful preparation and a heightened safety awareness.

Each type of hiking offers a unique set of experiences, challenges, and rewards, catering to the wide-ranging interests and abilities of the hiking community. Whether you're looking for a casual stroll in the woods, a rigorous trek through remote wilderness, or anything in between, a type of hiking will meet your needs. As the popularity of hiking continues to grow, so does the diversity of hiking experiences available, ensuring that the call of the trail is accessible to all who seek it.

The Physical and Mental Benefits

Hiking, often celebrated for its accessibility and connection to nature, offers many benefits beyond walking outdoors. These physical and mental benefits contribute to an individual's overall well-being, making hiking a recreational activity and a potent form of exercise and mental health therapy.

Physical Health Benefits

- **Cardiovascular and Respiratory Health:** Hiking is an excellent cardiovascular workout that helps strengthen the heart, lower blood pressure, and reduce the risk of heart disease. The varied terrain and elevation changes encountered on trails provide a natural interval training session, improving cardiovascular resilience and lung capacity.

- **Muscle Strength and Tone:** Hiking engages multiple muscle groups, including the quadriceps, hamstrings, glutes, and calves, increasing muscle strength and tone. Hiking uphill, in particular, is a powerful leg workout, while carrying a backpack adds resistance training for the upper body, enhancing core strength and stability.

- **Weight Management:** Hiking is an effective way to burn calories and manage weight. The number of calories burned depends on an individual's weight, the weight of the pack, and the hike's difficulty. On average, a person can burn between 400 and 600 calories per hour while hiking, making it an excellent activity for those looking to lose or maintain a healthy weight.

- **Bone Density:** Hiking is a weight-bearing exercise that forces you to work against gravity. This exercise strengthens bones, increasing bone density and reducing the risk of osteoporosis. The dynamic nature of hiking, with its varied terrain, also improves bone health more effectively than uniform surface exercises.

- **Balance and Coordination:** Trails' uneven surfaces and natural obstacles challenge hikers to maintain balance and coordination. Navigating rocks, roots, and uneven ground enhances proprioception (sense of body position) and improves overall balance and coordination, reducing the risk of falls and injuries in daily life.

Mental Health Benefits

- **Stress Reduction:** Hiking has been proven to significantly reduce stress levels and alleviate symptoms of anxiety and depression. Combining physical exercise, which releases endorphins (natural mood elevators), and the calming effects of being in nature creates a powerful antidote to stress. The outdoors's sights, sounds, and smells stimulate the senses, helping distract from daily worries and allowing a mental reset.

- **Improved Mood and Well-being:** Regular hikers often report improving their overall mood and well-being. This is attributed to the endorphins released during physical activity and the increased exposure to sunlight, which can boost serotonin levels, a mood-enhancing chemical in the brain. Hiking provides a sense of accomplishment and satisfaction, enhancing mood and self-esteem.

- **Enhanced Creativity and Problem-Solving:** Studies have shown that spending time in nature and engaging in physical activity like hiking can boost creativity and problem-solving skills by up to 50%. The natural environment stimulates the brain differently than urban environments, reducing mental fatigue and encouraging creative thought. Walking has been linked to a more fluid generation of ideas, making hiking an excellent activity for those seeking creative inspiration or solutions to problems.

- **Mindfulness and Meditation:** Hiking offers a unique opportunity for mindfulness and meditation. The rhythmic nature of walking, combined with the immersive sensory experience of being in nature, encourages a state of mindfulness—being fully present in the moment. Many hikers find that this focused attention on the present moment and their surroundings provides a form of moving meditation, enhancing mental clarity and emotional stability.

- **Social Connection:** While not exclusively a mental health benefit, the social aspect of hiking can significantly impact mental well-being. Hiking with others can strengthen relationships, provide a sense of community, and reduce feelings of loneliness and isolation. Group hikes and hiking clubs offer a way to connect with like-minded individuals, share experiences, and create lasting bonds.

Long-Term Mental Health Benefits

The long-term mental health benefits of hiking cannot be overstated. Regular engagement with this activity can improve stress management, mood regulation, and overall mental resilience. Hikers often report a greater sense of peace, satisfaction with life, and a deeper connection to nature, contributing to a positive mental outlook and enhanced life satisfaction.

Moreover, the challenges faced and overcome on the trail—navigating rugged terrain, completing a long-distance hike, or simply conquering personal fears—build confidence and a sense of achievement. These experiences translate into other areas of life, fostering a can-do attitude and resilience in facing challenges.

The physical and mental benefits of hiking are vast and well-documented, offering compelling reasons for individuals to lace up their boots and hit the trail. From improving cardiovascular health and muscle strength to reducing stress and enhancing creativity, hiking is a holistic activity that nurtures the body and mind. This overall positive impact on health and well-being can make individuals feel more energized and balanced, whether they undertake the journey alone or with a group.

Understanding Hiking - Hiking as a Form of Eco-Tourism

In the contemporary lexicon of travel, eco-tourism has emerged as a crucial concept, advocating for responsible travel to natural areas that conserves the environment, sustains the well-being of the local people, and involves interpretation and education. Within this paradigm, hiking represents a quintessential form of eco-tourism, embodying the principles of minimal environmental impact, support for conservation efforts, and promoting a deeper understanding and appreciation for nature among travelers.

Hiking and Eco-Tourism: A Natural Synergy

Hiking, at its core, is an activity that encourages immersion in the natural world with minimal resource use and a low carbon footprint. Unlike many forms of tourism, which rely on heavy infrastructure and can lead to significant environmental degradation, hiking necessitates little more than a trail. This simplicity and low impact make hiking an ideal eco-tourism activity, aligning with the goals of preserving nature while allowing people to experience and appreciate its beauty. The ease and accessibility of hiking can make individuals feel empowered to engage in eco-tourism.

The Benefits of Hiking for Eco-Tourism

- **Conservation Awareness and Support:** Hiking as eco-tourism fosters a direct connection between people and the natural environment, often inspiring a profound respect and a desire to protect natural landscapes. Hikers become advocates for conservation, supporting national parks, wilderness areas, and conservation efforts financially and through volunteer work. The presence of hikers also provides a subtle form of surveillance against illegal activities, such as poaching or logging, simply by their presence in remote areas.

- **Sustainable Economic Development:** Hiking contributes to sustainable economic development by providing a source of income that supports the local economy without compromising the environment. The influx of hikers benefits local guides, accommodations, and other small businesses, creating jobs and supporting the community while encouraging the preservation of natural areas as valuable resources.

- **Education and Cultural Exchange:** Eco-tourism, including hiking, offers significant opportunities for education and cultural exchange. Hikers learn about local flora and fauna, geology, and conservation challenges through interpretive signage, guided walks, and educational programs. Additionally, interaction with local communities allows for meaningful cultural exchange, fostering understanding and respect for different ways of life and traditional land stewardship practices.

Challenges of Hiking as Eco-Tourism

While hiking epitomizes eco-tourism, it is not without its challenges. As hiking's popularity grows, so do the pressures on natural areas, potentially leading to overcrowding, trail erosion, wildlife disturbance, and pollution. Managing these impacts requires careful planning and regulation by conservation authorities and responsible behavior from hikers.

- **Trail Management and Overcrowding:** Popular hiking destinations can suffer from overcrowding, especially during peak seasons, leading to trail degradation, litter, and other environmental impacts. Implementing quota systems, requiring permits, and promoting off-peak and lesser-known trails are strategies to manage these issues.

- **Responsible Hiker Behavior:** The Leave No Trace principles provide guidelines for minimizing the environmental impact of hiking. These include practices such as packing out all trash, staying on marked trails, respecting wildlife, and minimizing campfire impacts. However, it's not just about knowing these principles but also about adhering to them. Education and enforcement are vital in ensuring that hikers understand the gravity of their actions and adhere to these principles, thereby preserving the natural beauty of these areas.

Best Practices for Hiking as Eco-Tourism

For hiking to effectively fulfill its role as a form of eco-tourism, both hikers and the entities managing hiking destinations must adopt best practices prioritizing sustainability and conservation.

- **Supporting Conservation Efforts:** Hikers are not just visitors but active contributors to the conservation of these natural areas. They are supporting these vital conservation efforts by hiking in areas that channel funds directly into environmental protection, such as national parks or nature reserves. Volunteering for trail maintenance or conservation projects is another way hikers can give back and make a tangible difference.

- **Choosing Sustainable Gear:** Opting for eco-friendly, durable hiking gear reduces the environmental impact of manufacturing and disposing of equipment. Many outdoor brands are committed to sustainability, offering products made from recycled materials or designed with minimal environmental impact.

- **Respecting Local Communities:** Engaging with local communities respectfully and meaningfully is a cornerstone of eco-tourism. This includes hiring local guides, staying in locally owned accommodations, purchasing local products, and ensuring that hiking tourism's economic benefits are equitably distributed.

- **Educational Engagement:** Hikers should seek to learn about the places they visit, including their ecological, cultural, and historical significance. This knowledge deepens the hiking experience and fosters a greater appreciation and commitment to conservation.

Hiking is a prime example of eco-tourism, offering a sustainable way to explore and appreciate the natural world. It embodies the principles of environmental stewardship, economic sustainability, and cultural respect. However, the success of hiking as eco-tourism hinges on hikers' commitment to responsible practices and the effective management of natural areas to ensure they remain vibrant and accessible for future generations. By embracing the ethos of eco-tourism, hikers can ensure that their footprints on the trail contribute to preserving and appreciating the planet's invaluable natural heritage.

Dear Reader,

Thank you for reading "Two Paths Diverged – The Highs, Lows, and Hows Of Hiking."

As an independent author, your support means everything to me. If you enjoyed reading these pages, please consider leaving a review on the platform where you purchased it. Your feedback is invaluable and helps other readers discover this book.

Your honest review encourages me and helps me grow as a writer. Whether you loved it, found it thought-provoking, or have constructive criticism to share, I genuinely appreciate your input.

To leave a review, scan the QR code below to be taken to the Amazon page. Just a minute of your time and consideration are greatly appreciated.

Again, thank you for being a part of this literary adventure. I am honored.

     Sincerely,
       Brian Eby

CHAPTER

THREE

PREPARING FOR THE HIKE - PHYSICAL PREPARATION AND CONDITIONING

Embarking on a hiking adventure requires more than a strong will and a good pair of boots; it necessitates a foundation of physical preparation and conditioning to ensure safety, enjoyment, and the ability to meet the demands of the trail. Whether you're planning a leisurely day hike or a challenging multi-day trek, the following guidelines will help you physically prepare for the journey ahead.

Understanding the Demands of Hiking

Hiking can vary significantly in intensity, depending on the terrain, elevation gain, and trail distance. It's a full-body activity that primarily engages the leg muscles but also requires core stability and upper-body strength, especially when carrying a backpack. Additionally, outdoor trails' uneven and often unpredictable nature demands balance and flexibility to navigate obstacles and prevent injuries. Recognizing these demands is the first step in tailoring your physical preparation to meet the challenges of your planned hikes.

Building Endurance

Endurance is the most crucial aspect of physical preparation for hiking. It enables you to sustain prolonged physical activity and cover distances on the trail without undue fatigue.

- **Cardiovascular Training:** Incorporate aerobic exercises such as walking, running, cycling, or swimming into your routine. Start with sessions of at least 30 minutes, 3-4 times a week, gradually increasing the duration and intensity as your fitness improves. Aim to mimic the conditions of your hike by including hill work or stair climbing to better prepare for elevation gains.

- **Consistency and Progression:** Consistency in your training regimen is critical to building endurance. Gradually increase your training volume and intensity, following the principle of progressive overload to challenge your body and improve your aerobic capacity.

Strengthening Muscles

Strong muscles are essential for hiking, providing the power to ascend hills and the endurance for long distances. Focus on exercises that target the legs, core, and upper body.

- **Leg Strength:** Squats, lunges, step-ups, and leg presses will strengthen the quadriceps, hamstrings, glutes, and calves. Incorporating weighted or resistance-based exercises can simulate the effort required to hike with a backpack.

- **Core Stability:** A strong core maintains balance and stability on uneven terrain. Exercise like planks, bridges, abdominal crunches, and rotational movements to build a robust core.

- **Upper Body Strength:** While hiking is predominantly a lower-body activity, upper body strength is crucial for supporting a backpack and using trekking poles. Incorporate exercises such as push-ups, rows, and shoulder presses into your routine.

Enhancing Balance and Flexibility

Balance and flexibility are critical for navigating the variable and often rugged terrain encountered on hikes.

- **Balance Training:** Practice balance exercises such as single leg stands, Bosu ball exercises, or yoga poses to improve stability and coordination. Balance training helps prevent falls and injuries, especially on uneven surfaces.

- **Flexibility Work:** Regular stretching or yoga can increase flexibility, improve range of motion, and decrease the risk of muscle strains and joint injuries. Focus on stretching the major muscle groups used in hiking, including the calves, thighs, hips, lower back, and shoulders.

Practical Training: Simulating Hiking Conditions

The best preparation for hiking is hiking itself. Regular hikes build physical endurance and strength and acclimate your body to the activity's specific demands.

- **Trail Hiking:** Whenever possible, train on trails that simulate the conditions of your planned hikes. Use these outings to practice pacing, test your gear, and refine your technique, such as using trekking poles.

- **Weighted Hikes:** Practice hiking with a weighted backpack to prepare for backpacking or long-distance hikes. Start with a lighter load, gradually increasing the weight as you become more comfortable.

- **Cross-Training:** Incorporate cross-training activities that complement hiking, such as rock climbing for upper body strength and balance or paddle sports for core stability and endurance.

Listening to Your Body and Rest

As important as it is to push yourself in training, listening to your body and allowing adequate rest is equally crucial. Overtraining can lead to burnout, injury, and decreased performance. Incorporate rest days into your training schedule, and be attentive to signs of overexertion, such as prolonged muscle soreness, fatigue, or decreased motivation.

Nutrition and Hydration

Proper nutrition and hydration play a significant role in your physical preparation and performance on the trail. A balanced diet rich in nutrients supports muscle growth, repair, and overall energy levels. Hydrating effectively before, during, and after hikes is critical to maintain endurance and prevent dehydration.

Physical preparation and conditioning are foundational to a successful and enjoyable hiking experience. Hikers can significantly enhance their performance and resilience on the trail by building endurance, strength, balance, and flexibility and simulating hiking conditions through practical training. Remember, the goal of preparation is to endure the hike and enjoy it fully, embracing the challenges and rewards of the journey with confidence and vitality.

Preparing for the Hike - Essential Gear and How to Select It

A successful and enjoyable hiking experience begins with the right gear. It is critical to equip yourself with essential items that are reliable, comfortable, and suited to the conditions you will face.

Footwear: The Foundation of Every Hike

- **Types of Footwear:** Hiking footwear ranges from lightweight trail shoes to sturdy hiking and mountaineering boots. The right choice depends on the terrain, the weight you'll carry, and your preference for ankle support.

- **Selection Tips:** Look for shoes with good traction, support, and waterproof features. Ensure a comfortable fit by trying them on in the afternoon (feet swell throughout the day) and wearing the socks you plan to hike in. Consider the break-in period for heavier boots.

Backpacks: Carrying Your Essentials

- **Types of Backpacks:** Daypacks are suitable for short hikes, while overnight and extended-trip backpacks, which range from 30 to 80+ liters, are necessary for carrying additional gear and provisions.

- **Selection Tips:** Look for a backpack with an ergonomic design that distributes weight evenly across your hips and shoulders. The key features include adjustable straps, a padded back panel, and sufficient compartments for organization. Fit is crucial—ensure the backpack matches your torso length and hip width.

Clothing: Dressing for Success

- **Layering System:** Effective hiking attire follows a three-layer system: a moisture-wicking base layer, an insulating middle layer, and a waterproof and breathable outer layer. This system keeps you dry, warm, and protected from the elements.

- **Selection Tips:** Choose materials that provide comfort, breathability, and moisture-wicking properties, such as merino wool or synthetic fibers. Avoid cotton, as it retains moisture. For the outer layer, look for durable water-repellent (DWR) coatings and taped seams for enhanced waterproofing.

Navigation Tools: Staying on Course

- **Essential Navigation Tools:** A map and compass are indispensable for wilderness hiking, even if you plan to use a GPS device or smartphone app. They require no power and work in areas where electronic devices might fail.

- **Selection Tips:** Ensure your map is up-to-date and covers the area you'll be hiking in. Learn how to use a compass alongside a map for accurate navigation. Consider waterproof cases or laminated maps for durability.

First Aid Kit: Preparedness for Emergencies

- **Kit Essentials:** A hiking first aid kit should include items to treat cuts, blisters, burns, and other minor injuries. It should also include personal medications, an emergency blanket, and items for tick removal and insect bites.

- **Selection Tips:** Tailor your first aid kit to the length of your hike and your group size. Waterproof containers keep contents dry. Familiarize yourself with the use of each item in the kit.

Hydration Systems: Staying Hydrated

- **Hydration Options:** Water bottles and hydration reservoirs are the main water-carrying options. Reservoirs offer convenience through a drink tube, allowing for easy access without stopping.

- **Selection Tips:** When deciding how much water to carry, consider the duration of your hike and the availability of water sources. Look for durable, leak-proof bottles and reservoirs with easy-to-clean openings.

Nutrition: Fueling Your Body

- **Food Selection:** Opt for high-energy, lightweight, and non-perishable foods. Energy bars, trail mix, dried fruits, and jerky are excellent choices. For longer hikes, consider dehydrated meals that only require hot water.

- **Selection Tips:** Balance nutrition and taste preferences. Pack a little extra as a safety margin. Remember to plan for efficient waste disposal, such as resealable bags to pack trash.

Lighting: Illuminating Your Path

- **Lighting Gear:** A reliable headlamp is essential for any hike, providing hands-free convenience. Look for models with adjustable brightness settings and a red-light mode to preserve night vision.

- **Selection Tips:** Check the lumens (light output) and battery life. For versatility, consider headlamps with rechargeable batteries or the ability to use both rechargeable and disposable batteries.

Shelter: Protection from the Elements

- **Shelter Options:** A lightweight emergency bivvy or space blanket may be sufficient for day hikes. Overnight hikes require a tent or hammock with appropriate rain protection and bug netting.

- **Selection Tips:** Consider the tent's weight, seasonality (3-season vs. 4-season), and capacity. Ensure it's easy to set up and offers adequate ventilation to prevent condensation.

Multi-Tool and Repair Kits: Readiness for Repairs

- **Essential Tools:** A multi-tool with a knife, pliers, and screwdrivers can be invaluable for repairs and unexpected needs. Pack a small repair kit with duct tape, zip ties, and spare gear parts.

- **Selection Tips:** Choose a lightweight yet durable multi-tool. Tailor your repair kit to your gear and know how to use each item.

Selecting the right gear for hiking involves balancing functionality, weight, and personal preferences. Start with the essentials listed here, and refine your kit based on experiences and the specific demands of your hikes. Remember, the goal is to enjoy the outdoors safely and comfortably; the right gear is vital. Always test new gear on short hikes before embarking on longer adventures to ensure it meets your needs and expectations.

Embarking on a hiking adventure demands physical preparation, the right gear, and careful consideration of your nutrition and hydration needs. Proper nutrition fuels your body for the exertion of hiking, while adequate hydration is crucial for maintaining peak performance and preventing heat-related illnesses.

Understanding Your Nutritional Needs

When planning for a hike, it's essential to understand the energy your body requires. Hiking can burn anywhere from 300 to 600 calories per hour, depending on factors like your weight, backpack weight, and the hike's difficulty. Your body needs a balance of carbohydrates, proteins, and fats to sustain energy, repair muscles, and maintain body functions.

Carbohydrates

Carbohydrates are your body's primary energy source during high-intensity activities like hiking. They're quickly broken down into glucose, fueling your muscles and brain. Prioritize complex carbohydrates such as whole grains, fruits, and vegetables, which provide sustained energy release, and include some simple carbohydrates like energy gels or dried fruit for quick energy boosts.

Proteins

Proteins are essential for muscle repair and recovery, especially on multi-day hikes. Include lean protein sources such as nuts, seeds, jerky, and legumes in your hiking diet. For longer hikes, consider protein-rich meal replacements or supplements to ensure adequate intake.

Fats

Fats are a dense energy source, making them invaluable for long-duration activities. They provide essential fatty acids and help absorb fat-soluble vitamins. Incorporate healthy fats in nuts, seeds, avocados, and olive oil into your meals and snacks.

Planning Your Meals and Snacks

Proper meal planning is crucial to meeting your nutritional needs while minimizing pack weight and waste. Plan meals and snacks that are nutrient-dense, lightweight, and easy to prepare.

Breakfast

Start your day with a hearty breakfast with complex carbohydrates, protein, and healthy fats to fuel your morning hike. Options like oatmeal with nuts and dried fruits, whole-grain tortillas with nut butter, or high-protein granola bars are excellent choices.

Lunch and Dinner

For midday and evening meals, focus on replenishing spent energy and providing nutrients for muscle recovery. Portable, non-perishable items like whole-grain wraps, dehydrated meals, tuna packets, and ready-to-eat rice are convenient and satisfying. Incorporate dried vegetables and spices to enhance flavor and nutrient content.

Snacks

Snacks are vital for maintaining energy levels between meals. Pack a variety of snacks such as trail mix, energy bars, fruit leathers, and nut butters. These provide a quick and easy way to consume calories and nutrients without stopping for a complete meal.

Hydration Strategies

Hydration is equally as crucial as nutrition. Dehydration can lead to decreased performance, fatigue, and heat-related severe illnesses. Understanding and implementing effective hydration strategies is critical to a successful hiking experience.

Water Intake Guidelines

The amount of water needed varies by individual and conditions. Still, a general guideline is to drink about half a liter (17 ounces) of water every hour of moderate activity in moderate temperatures. This amount should increase in hotter conditions or for more strenuous hikes.

Electrolyte Balance

Sweat loss during hiking includes water and electrolytes, which are critical for muscle function and hydration. Use electrolyte replacement solutions, tablets, or powders to replenish sodium, potassium, magnesium, and calcium. These can be added to water or consumed in electrolyte-rich foods.

Hydration Systems

Choose a hydration system that suits your preference and the length of your hike. Options include water bottles, hydration bladders with a drinking hose, or water filtration systems for accessing natural water sources. Always start with a total water supply and know the location of water sources on longer trails.

Tips for Eating and Drinking on the Trail

Eating and drinking regularly on the trail can be challenging, especially during rigorous hikes. Here are some tips to help manage your nutrition and hydration:

- **Eat Small, Frequent Meals and Snacks:** Consuming smaller amounts of food more frequently can help maintain energy levels without weighing you down.

- **Prioritize Convenience:** Pack foods that are easy to eat on the go and require minimal preparation.

- **Stay ahead of Hunger and Thirst: Don't wait until you're starving or parched to eat or drink—by then, you'll already be** depleting your reserves.

- **Adjust Based on Conditions:** Increase your calorie and fluid intake in cold or hot weather to match your body's increased needs.

Pre-Hike and Post-Hike Nutrition

What you eat before and after your hike can significantly impact your performance and recovery.

- **Pre-Hike:** Consume a meal or snack rich in complex carbohydrates 1-2 hours before hiking to ensure your energy stores are topped up.

- **Post-Hike:** Focus on recovery by eating a meal rich in protein and carbohydrates within two hours after your hike to replenish energy stores and aid muscle repair.

Special Considerations

- **Altitude:** Hiking at high altitudes increases fluid loss and energy expenditure. To combat altitude sickness and maintain energy, increase your water intake and consume more calories, mainly carbohydrates.

- **Dietary Restrictions:** Plan accordingly for specific dietary needs or restrictions. Many trail-friendly foods cater to various dietary preferences, including vegan, gluten-free, and allergy-friendly options.

Proper nutrition and hydration are the cornerstones of a successful hiking experience. By understanding and addressing your body's needs, you can ensure sustained energy, optimal performance, and overall enjoyment of your hiking adventures. Remember, every hiker's needs differ, so listening to your body and adjusting your nutrition and hydration plan is essential. With careful planning and mindful consumption, you can confidently tackle any trail, knowing you're well-fueled for the journey ahead.

Necessary Skills

The Basics of Map Reading

Maps are fundamental tools for navigation, offering a representation of the physical environment on a manageable scale. Understanding how to read a map is crucial.

- **Types of Maps:** Familiarize yourself with topographic maps, which show terrain features, elevation, landmarks, and trail maps specific to hiking areas. Each type provides different details essential for navigation.

- **Map Symbols and Legend:** Learn to interpret map symbols and the legend, which explain the meaning of colors, shapes, and lines, representing various physical features like trails, rivers, and elevation contours.

- **Scale and Distance:** Understanding the map's scale allows you to estimate distances. This knowledge is vital for planning your hike and estimating travel times.

- **Contour Lines:** Contour lines indicate elevation and the shape of the terrain. Closely spaced lines signify steep slopes, while widely spaced lines indicate gentler slopes. Mastery of reading contour lines enables hikers to visualize the terrain ahead and choose the best path.

Compass Skills

A compass is a powerful navigation tool when used with a map. It points to magnetic north, helping hikers orient themselves and their maps to the surrounding landscape.

- **Basic Compass Features:** Learn the parts of a compass, including the magnetic needle, orienting arrow, baseplate, and rotating bezel.

- **Orienting a Map:** Use a compass to align your map with the landscape. This involves rotating the map and compass until the magnetic needle aligns with the map's north.

- **Taking Bearings:** A bearing is a direction or path between two points. To navigate using bearings, determine the bearing from your location to your destination with your compass, then follow that direction in the terrain.

- **Triangulation:** Triangulation is used to pinpoint your location by taking bearings from two or more known landmarks and drawing lines on your map that intersect at your position.

GPS and Electronic Navigation

Global Positioning System (GPS) devices and smartphones with GPS capabilities have become popular tools for outdoor navigation, offering convenience and real-time data.

- **GPS Devices:** Handheld GPS devices can provide precise location information, display maps, and allow users to mark waypoints and track their routes. Learn to use features specific to hiking, such as setting waypoints, following a predetermined route, and marking points of interest.

- **Smartphone Apps:** Various apps turn smartphones into practical navigation tools. Choose apps designed for outdoor activities, offering downloadable maps, trail databases, and route-planning tools. Remember that relying solely on electronic devices is risky due to potential battery failure or lack of signal. Always carry a map and compass as backups.

Navigating Without a Compass or GPS

In situations where you find yourself without modern navigation tools, natural navigation methods can provide guidance.

- **Using the Sun:** The sun rises in the east and sets in the west, providing an essential directional guide. Shadows can also help determine direction based on the time of day.

- **Stars:** Familiarize yourself with constellations like the Big Dipper and Orion, which can help orient you at night. The North Star (Polaris) in the Northern Hemisphere indicates true north.

- **Landmarks:** Use natural and artificial landmarks to navigate. Mountains, rivers, and distinct trees can serve as reference points to maintain your bearings.

Practical Navigation Tips

Applying navigation skills in real-world scenarios requires practice and attention to detail.

- **Plan Your Route:** Plan your route using a map before heading out. Identify landmarks, calculate distances, and note potential challenges.

- **Stay Oriented:** Regularly check your position against the map and surroundings. This habit prevents disorientation and ensures you're on the right track.

- **Pacing and Timing:** Learn to estimate distances by pacing and timing your travel. This skill helps gauge how far you've traveled and how far you have to go.

- **Buddy System:** Designate navigation tasks for different group members when hiking. This approach fosters teamwork and ensures that more than one person is proficient in navigation.

- **Leave No Trace:** As you navigate, practice Leave No Trace principles to minimize environmental impact. Stick to established trails where possible and avoid disturbing wildlife.

Advanced Navigation Techniques

Consider advanced techniques and training for those looking to enhance their navigation skills.

- **Night Navigation:** Practice navigating by the stars and in low-light conditions. This skill is invaluable for unexpected overnight stays or early starts.

- **Off-Trail Navigation:** Navigating areas without established trails requires a deep understanding of terrain reading and compass work. It's recommended only for experienced hikers with advanced skills.

- **Navigation Courses:** Many organizations offer wilderness navigation courses. These courses provide hands-on experience, practical exercises, and expert instruction to sharpen your skills.

Mastering navigation is a journey that enhances your hiking experience, safety, and independence in the wilderness. Start with foundational skills like map reading and compass use, then gradually incorporate GPS technology and natural navigation methods into your repertoire. Practice regularly, starting with more straightforward hikes to build confidence and competence. Remember, the best navigators blend preparation, skill, and respect for the environment to explore the natural world responsibly and safely. Whether following a well-marked trail or forging your path, navigation skills are crucial to unlocking your outdoor adventures' full potential.

Hiking through nature's vast and varied landscapes offers unparalleled experiences and adventures. However, with the beauty and solitude of the wild come inherent risks that every hiker must recognize and manage. Understanding and mitigating these risks is essential for a safe and enjoyable outdoor experience.

Environmental Hazards

While often stunningly beautiful, the natural environment can pose significant risks to hikers. From unpredictable weather to challenging terrain, hikers must be prepared to face and navigate various hazards.

Weather Conditions

- **Preparation:** Check weather forecasts and understand the implications of weather changes in your specific hiking area. Conditions in mountainous areas, for example, can shift rapidly from sunny to stormy.

- **Mitigation:** Carry appropriate gear for potential weather conditions, including rain gear, extra layers for cold, and sun protection. Learn the signs of approaching storms and hypothermia so you can take action early.

Terrain Challenges

- **Preparation:** Research your hiking route to understand the terrain. Be aware of steep inclines, river crossings, and areas prone to rockslides or avalanches.

- **Mitigation:** Use appropriate footwear with good traction and ankle support. Carry trekking poles for additional stability. Consider specialized equipment like crampons for ice or a life jacket for water crossings in areas with unique terrain challenges.

Altitude Sickness

- **Preparation:** Altitude sickness can affect anyone ascending above 2,500 meters (8,200 feet). Understand the symptoms, which include headache, nausea, and fatigue.

- **Mitigation:** Acclimatize gradually to higher altitudes, increasing sleeping elevation by no more than 300-500 meters (1,000-1,600 feet) per day. Stay hydrated and consider descending if symptoms worsen.

Wildlife Encounters

Wildlife encounters, often a highlight of hiking, can become risky if not managed properly. Respect for wildlife and knowledge of how to behave in their presence are crucial.

Bears

- **Preparation:** Learn about bear activity in the area. Carry bear spray where permitted, and know how to use it.

- **Mitigation:** Make noise while hiking to avoid surprising bears. Store food and scented items properly using bear-proof containers or techniques. Never approach or feed wildlife.

Snakes and Insects

- **Preparation:** Identify potentially dangerous snakes and insects in the area. Wear long pants and closed shoes to protect against bites and stings.

- **Mitigation:** Stay on trails to minimize the risk of snake bites. Use insect repellent and check for ticks regularly. Learn the first aid response for bites and stings.

Getting Lost

One of the most common risks while hiking is getting lost, especially on remote or poorly marked trails.

- **Preparation:** Carry a map, compass, and GPS device. Know how to use them to navigate your route.

- **Mitigation:** Stay on marked trails, pay attention to trail markers, and regularly check your position against your map. If you realize you're lost, stay calm, stay put if safe, and use the STOP acronym: Stop, Think, Observe, Plan.

Personal Safety Measures

Personal preparedness is the foundation of risk management in hiking. This includes physical preparation, emergency planning, and carrying essential gear.

Physical Fitness

- **Preparation:** Tailor your hiking plans to your physical fitness level. Train for your hike by gradually increasing your endurance and strength.

- **Mitigation:** Listen to your body, take breaks, and be willing to turn back if the hike becomes too challenging.

Emergency Planning

- **Preparation:** Inform someone of your hike itinerary and expected return time. Research the area to know the location of emergency services.

- **Mitigation:** Carry a basic first aid kit, know how to signal for help, and have a plan for emergencies, such as sudden illness or injury.

Essential Gear

- **Preparation:** Pack the "Ten Essentials" for hiking, including navigation tools, sun protection, insulation, illumination, first-aid supplies, fire-making tools, repair kit, nutrition, hydration, and emergency shelter.

- **Mitigation:** Know how to use each piece of your gear. Regularly check your equipment before each hike to ensure it's in good working condition.

Group Dynamics

Hiking in groups can add a layer of safety but also requires additional considerations.

- **Preparation:** Ensure all group members are informed about the hike, including its difficulty and potential risks. Establish clear communication and decision-making processes.

- **Mitigation:** Stay together, adapting the hike's pace to the slowest member. Have a plan for what to do if the group gets separated.

Hiking invites us to explore and enjoy the natural world, but it also demands respect for the environment and awareness of the risks involved. By understanding and proactively managing these risks, hikers can significantly enhance their safety and enjoyment on the trail. Preparation, knowledge, and caution are the keys to a successful hiking adventure, allowing us to experience the wonders of nature with confidence and security. Remember, the goal is to reach the destination and do so safely, preserving our well-being and the beauty of the wilderness we set out to explore.

Essential First Aid

Assessing the Situation

- **Scene Safety:** Before approaching an injured person, ensure the scene is safe for both the rescuer and the victim. Look for hazards like falling rocks, unstable ground, or wild animals.

- **Primary Assessment:** Check for responsiveness, airway blockages, breathing, and circulation. This quick assessment helps identify life-threatening conditions.

Common Injuries and Conditions

Cuts and Scrapes

- **Care:** Clean the wound with clean water to remove debris. Apply gentle pressure with a sterile dressing to stop bleeding. Once bleeding is controlled, apply an antibiotic ointment and cover with a bandage.

- **Prevention:** Wear appropriate protective clothing and be mindful of the terrain to avoid falls and scratches.

Sprains and Strains

- **Care:** Use the RICE method—rest, Ice, Compression, and Elevation. Rest the injured limb, apply ice to reduce swelling, use a bandage for compression, and keep the limb elevated.

- **Prevention:** Wear appropriate footwear and use trekking poles for stability.

Fractures

- **Care:** Immobilize the injured area with a splint. Avoid moving the person unless necessary. Seek emergency help.

- **Prevention:** Be cautious when navigating rugged terrain.

Heat Exhaustion and Heatstroke

- **Care for Heat Exhaustion:** Move the person to a cooler place, remove excess clothing, and give cool water to drink.

- **Care for Heatstroke:** This is a medical emergency. Cool the person rapidly with whatever means available and seek emergency help immediately.

- **Prevention:** Stay hydrated, wear appropriate clothing, and avoid hiking during the hottest part of the day.

Hypothermia

- **Care:** Remove wet clothing and replace it with dry, warm layers. Warm the core body first, not the extremities, which can shock the heart. Provide warm, non-alcoholic beverages if the person is conscious.

- **Prevention:** Dress in layers, stay dry, and understand the signs of hypothermia.

Dehydration

- **Care:** Prevent dehydration by encouraging regular fluid intake, even before feeling thirsty. Treat mild dehydration by resting and drinking water or sports drinks.

- **Prevention:** Carry and drink water regularly and avoid diuretics such as caffeine and alcohol.

Altitude Sickness

- **Care:** Descend to a lower altitude if symptoms worsen. Keep the person warm and hydrated.

- **Prevention:** Ascend gradually to allow time for acclimatization, and consider spending a few days at a moderate altitude before going higher.

When to Seek Further Medical Help

- **Severe Injuries:** Compound fractures, deep wounds with uncontrollable bleeding, or head injuries require immediate medical attention.

- **Persistent Symptoms:** If symptoms of altitude sickness, dehydration, hypothermia, or heat-related illnesses do not improve with initial care, seek medical help.

- **Loss of Consciousness:** Any loss of consciousness, even briefly, warrants a medical evaluation.

Wilderness First Aid Courses

A wilderness first aid course is highly recommended for those who frequently hike or embark on outdoor adventures. These courses are specifically designed to provide hands-on training for managing medical emergencies in remote settings where immediate professional medical help may not be available.

While a comprehensive exploration of first aid and emergency medical procedures for hiking could fill volumes, this overview highlights the importance of preparedness and basic care knowledge. Carrying a well-stocked first aid kit and possessing the skills to use it can make a significant difference in managing common injuries and conditions on the trail. Remember, the best approach to outdoor safety combines prevention, preparation, and informed action.

Trail Etiquette

Trail etiquette encompasses the unwritten rules and behaviors that ensure hiking experiences are enjoyable, safe, and environmentally sustainable for everyone. Understanding and adhering to these guidelines fosters a sense of community among hikers and helps protect the natural landscapes we cherish.

Right-of-Way on the Trail

Navigating encounters with other hikers, cyclists, and equestrians on the trail is fundamental to trail etiquette, requiring awareness and courtesy.

- **Hikers vs. Bikers:** Generally, bikers are expected to yield to hikers. However, because bikes often move faster and require more effort to stop and start, it's courteous for hikers to step aside when it is safe.

- **Hikers vs. Equestrians:** Hikers should yield to horseback riders. Horses can be easily startled, so it's advised to step off the trail on the downhill side (to appear less significant) and speak calmly to allow the horse to recognize you as human.

- **Uphill vs. Downhill Hikers:** Uphill hikers have the right-of-way. Climbing is more strenuous than descending, and stopping can break an uphill hiker's rhythm. Uphill hikers may step aside to catch their breath, offering downhill hikers the path.

Minimizing Environmental Impact

Following Leave No Trace principles is essential for preserving natural beauty and ecosystem health.

- **Stay on Designated Trails:** Venturing off-trail can cause erosion, disturb wildlife habitats, and harm plant life. Stick to marked paths unless in designated dispersed areas.

- **Pack It In, Pack It Out:** All garbage, including organic waste like fruit peels or nuts, should be carried out. Biodegradable items can still take years to decompose and may not be native to the ecosystem.

- **Proper Waste Disposal:** Human waste should be buried in a small hole 6-8 inches deep and at least 200 feet away from water sources, trails, and campgrounds. Use established toilets when available.

- **Respect Wildlife:** Observe animals from a distance, do not feed them, and store food securely to avoid attracting wildlife to human areas.

Respectful Interactions

The trail allows everyone to enjoy nature, find peace, and seek adventure. Respectful interactions ensure a positive experience for all.

- **Greeting Fellow Hikers:** A simple hello or nod acknowledges others and fosters a friendly atmosphere. Respect others' desire for solitude, recognizing when a brief acknowledgment suffices versus engaging in conversation.

- **Noise Levels:** Keep noise to a minimum to preserve the natural soundscape. Avoid loud music or voices. If you prefer music, use headphones at a volume that still allows you to hear your surroundings.

- **Pets on the Trail:** Keep dogs under control and on a leash where required. This protects wildlife, other hikers, and your pet. Always pack out pet waste.

- **Technology on the Trail:** Use electronic devices respectfully. If you take calls or listen to music, step aside from the trail and keep the volume low to minimize disturbances to wildlife and other hikers.

Camping Etiquette

For those venturing into overnight backpacking, additional considerations come into play to minimize impact and ensure safety.

- **Campsite Selection:** Use established campsites when available. If dispersed camping is allowed, choose a site that will not damage your stay. Avoid camping too close to water sources to protect riparian areas.

- **Campfires:** Follow local guidelines regarding campfires. Use existing fire rings, keep fires small, and ensure they are completely extinguished before leaving. Consider using a lightweight stove for cooking to reduce fire impact.

Managing Conflicts

Despite everyone's best efforts, conflicts can arise on the trail. It is vital to handle these situations with patience and diplomacy.

- **Addressing Issues:** If you encounter someone not adhering to trail etiquette or regulations, approach the situation calmly and kindly. Often, people are unaware rather than intentionally disrespectful.

- **Seeking Solutions:** Focus on finding a solution that respects all parties' safety and enjoyment. Sometimes, explaining the reasoning behind certain etiquette or rules can enlighten and resolve the conflict.

Trail etiquette is more than just following rules; it embodies a spirit of respect, responsibility, and stewardship towards nature and our fellow adventurers. By practicing these guidelines, hikers enhance their experience and contribute to a sustainable, enjoyable, and safe outdoor community. As we venture into the wild, let's carry the principles of courtesy, respect, and preservation, ensuring these cherished landscapes remain vibrant and accessible for generations.

The "Leave No Trace" (LNT) principles are guidelines developed by the Leave No Trace Center for Outdoor Ethics to promote outdoor conservation. These principles help hikers and outdoor enthusiasts minimize their impact on the natural environment, ensuring that wild places remain beautiful and untouched for future generations. Understanding and implementing these seven principles is crucial for anyone venturing into the great outdoors.

1. Plan and Prepare

Proper planning and preparation are crucial to minimizing your impact on the environment. This principle involves researching the area you plan to visit, understanding regulations and particular concerns, and preparing for extreme weather, hazards, and emergencies. It also means considering the size of your group and splitting larger parties into smaller groups to reduce foot traffic and environmental impact.

- **Why It Matters:** Adequate preparation reduces the likelihood of resource damage and ensures safety. By knowing the regulations and what to expect, you can avoid sensitive areas, pack necessary equipment to minimize waste, and reduce the risk of accidents.

2. Travel and Camp on Durable Surfaces

The goal here is to minimize damage to the land by sticking to established trails and campsites. Durable surfaces include established trails, rock, gravel, dry grasses, or snow. When camping, use sites that are already established whenever possible, and avoid altering sites for your tent.

- **Why It Matters:** Traveling and camping on durable surfaces reduces the creation of social trails, which can cause erosion and habitat destruction. It also helps preserve the area's natural beauty and ensures that wildlife habitats are not disturbed.

3. Dispose of Waste Properly

"Pack it in, pack it out" is the mantra here. All garbage, including food scraps and litter, should be packed out. When it comes to human waste, bury it in a 6-8 inches deep cat hole, at least 200 feet from water, trails, and campsites. To wash yourself or your dishes, carry water 200 feet away from streams or lakes and use small amounts of biodegradable soap.

- **Why It Matters:** Proper waste disposal keeps the environment clean, prevents pollution of water sources, and avoids attracting wildlife to human food.

4. Leave What You Find

Preserve the past: examine cultural or historic structures and artifacts, but do not touch them. Leave rocks, plants, and other natural objects as you find them. Avoid introducing or transporting non-native species by cleaning your boots before and after your trip to avoid spreading invasive species.

- **Why It Matters:** This principle helps maintain the wilderness's natural diversity and beauty. It also ensures that future visitors experience the same sense of discovery and awe.

5. Minimize Campfire Impacts

Campfires can cause lasting impacts on the environment. Use a lightweight stove for cooking and enjoy a candle lantern for light. Where fires are permitted, use established fire rings, keep fires small, and burn all wood and coals to ash. Put out fires completely and scatter cool ashes.

- **Why It Matters:** Minimizing campfire impacts reduces the risk of wildfires, preserves areas' natural appearance, and prevents the depletion of wood resources.

6. Respect Wildlife

Observe wildlife from a distance, and do not follow or approach them. Never feed animals, as doing so damages their health, alters natural behaviors, and exposes them to predators and other dangers. Protect wildlife and your food by storing rations and trash securely.

- **Why It Matters:** Respecting wildlife ensures that animals remain wild and unhabituated to human presence, reducing the risk of dangerous encounters and preserving natural ecosystems.

7. Be Considerate of Other Visitors

Respect other visitors and protect the quality of their experience. Be courteous on the trail and let nature's sounds prevail. Avoid loud voices and noises. Yield to other users on the trail and take breaks away from the trail to let others pass.

- **Why It Matters:** Being considerate of other visitors ensures that everyone can enjoy their outdoor experience without unnecessary disturbances. It promotes a sense of community and mutual respect among those sharing the wilderness.

Implementation in Hiking

Implementing the LNT principles while hiking contributes to preserving the environment and enhancing the experience for everyone. It involves making conscious decisions, from the planning stage to the execution of your hike, and adopting habits that respect the natural world.

Plan and Prepare by researching your hike and packing accordingly, ensuring you have the right equipment to Leave No Trace.

Travel and Camp on Durable Surfaces by sticking to trails and established campsites, avoiding virgin soil and vegetation.

Proper Waste disposal involves packing all trash, using bear cans or bags for food waste, and managing human waste responsibly.

Leave What You Find by taking only photos and leaving rocks, plants, and artifacts for others to enjoy.

Minimize Campfire Impacts by using stoves for cooking and respecting fire restrictions to prevent wildfires.

Respect Wildlife by keeping a safe distance, not feeding animals, and storing food securely to avoid attracting wildlife.

Be Considerate of Other Visitors by keeping noise levels down, yielding to other hikers, and ensuring your actions do not detract from others' experiences.

The Leave No Trace principles offer a framework for making ethical decisions in the outdoors. By adhering to these guidelines, hikers can significantly reduce their environmental impact and ensure that the wilderness remains pristine for future generations. Embracing these principles is a commitment to conservation, respect for wildlife, and consideration for fellow outdoor enthusiasts. As we venture into nature, let's carry the responsibility of leaving no trace, preserving the integrity and beauty of our natural world.

Respecting wildlife and preserving natural habitats are core tenets of responsible hiking and outdoor ethics. The wilderness offers us a unique escape, a chance to connect with the natural world away from the hustle of daily life. Yet, with this privilege comes the responsibility to protect and conserve the environment and its inhabitants.

Understanding the Impact of Human Presence

Humans inherently impact the environment they enter. Trails carve through habitats, and our mere presence can alter wildlife behavior. Animals may grow accustomed to human presence, altering their feeding, mating, and predatory behaviors, which can have cascading effects on the ecosystem.

The Importance of Minimizing Disturbance

Minimizing our disturbance helps maintain the natural balance and ensures that wildlife continues to thrive in their habitat. This involves staying quiet, keeping a respectful distance from animals, and not altering or damaging their environment.

Principles of Wildlife Respect

Observe from a Distance

Wildlife should be observed from a distance that doesn't alter their behavior. Use binoculars or zoom lenses to view and photograph animals without getting too close. Approaching wildlife can stress the animals, leading them to expend the energy they need to feed, care for their young, or stay warm.

Do Not Feed Wildlife

Feeding wildlife disrupts their natural diet and can lead to dependency on human-provided foods, malnutrition, and increased mortality rates. It also increases the likelihood of dangerous human-animal interactions.

Control Pets

Pets can harass or harm wildlife, even if unintentionally. Keeping pets on a leash and under control, or better yet, leaving them at home when visiting sensitive wildlife areas, helps protect both pets and wildlife.

Travel in Small Groups

Large groups are more likely to disturb wildlife and their habitats. Traveling in smaller groups reduces noise and disturbance, making it easier to manage the environmental impact.

Preserving Natural Habitats

Natural habitats are complex ecosystems that provide shelter, food, and breeding grounds for wildlife. Preserving these areas is essential for species' survival and the planet's overall health.

Stay on Designated Trails

Straying from established trails can trample vegetation, disturb wildlife, and contribute to erosion. By sticking to trails, hikers can minimize their impact on the surrounding habitat.

Practice Leave No Trace Principles

Adhering to the Leave No Trace principles, such as packing out all trash, camping on durable surfaces, and minimizing campfire impacts, helps preserve natural habitats. Each principle is designed to reduce human impact on the environment.

Participate in Conservation Efforts

Whether through volunteering, donating, or participating in citizen science projects, engaging in local conservation efforts can have a tangible impact on preserving natural habitats.

The Role of Education and Advocacy

Educating oneself and others about wildlife respect and habitat preservation is crucial for long-term conservation success. Hikers can become advocates for the environment by sharing knowledge, encouraging responsible behavior among peers, and supporting conservation-oriented policies and organizations.

Educate Fellow Hikers

Sharing knowledge about wildlife respect and habitat preservation with fellow hikers amplifies the message. Simple acts, like explaining why feeding wildlife is harmful or why staying on trails is essential, can influence behavior and foster a culture of conservation.

Support Conservation Organizations

Many organizations work tirelessly to protect natural habitats and wildlife. Supporting these organizations through donations, membership, or volunteering amplifies their efforts and contributes to broader conservation goals.

Advocate for Protection Policies

Advocating for policies and regulations that protect natural habitats and wildlife is another way hikers can contribute to conservation efforts. This can involve anything from participating in public comment periods for local conservation projects to supporting national or global environmental policies.

Ethical Photography and Social Media Sharing

In the age of social media, sharing experiences online has become a part of many hikers' adventures. However, it's essential to consider the impact of sharing locations and interactions with wildlife.

Share Responsibly

Consider the potential impact when posting photos or stories of wildlife and natural habitats. Avoid geotagging sensitive locations to prevent overcrowding and habitat degradation. Encourage respectful behavior by highlighting ethical practices in your posts.

Educate Through Social Media

Social media can be a powerful tool for conservation education. Use your platform to raise awareness about respecting wildlife and preserving habitats, sharing tips for responsible hiking and ethical wildlife observation.

The Ripple Effect of Responsible Hiking

Every action taken to respect wildlife and preserve natural habitats while hiking contributes to a more considerable effort to protect the planet's biodiversity. Responsible hiking practices create a ripple effect, influencing the immediate area visited and the broader conservation culture.

Fostering a Conservation Ethic

By embodying a conservation ethic in our hiking practices, we contribute to a cultural shift towards more outstanding environmental stewardship. This shift can influence policies, funding, and public awareness, leading to more significant conservation outcomes.

The Legacy of Respect and Preservation

The choices we make today shape the natural world for future generations. Through respectful interaction with wildlife and diligent efforts to preserve natural habitats, we leave a legacy of conservation that ensures the continued richness and diversity of the planet's ecosystems.

Respecting wildlife and preserving natural habitats while hiking are not just acts of individual responsibility but also contribute to a collective effort to protect and conserve the natural world. By understanding the impact of our actions, adhering to principles of respect and preservation, and advocating for conservation, hikers can enjoy the profound beauty and solace of the wilderness while ensuring it remains vibrant and intact for future explorers. As we lace up our boots and set out on the trail, let's commit deeply to the environment, embracing our role as stewards of the Earth's precious natural heritage.

Exploring the most famous hiking trails across the continents offers a glimpse into the diversity and beauty of the world's landscapes. Here are 15 iconic trails that capture the essence of adventure:

1. **Appalachian Trail, USA** - Spanning 2,200 miles across the Eastern United States, it offers hikers breathtaking views of the American wilderness.

2. **Pacific Crest Trail, USA**—This 2,650-mile journey from Mexico to Canada passes through California, Oregon, and Washington.

3. **Inca Trail, Peru** - This ancient trail winds through the Andes to the mystical ruins of Machu Picchu.

4. **Tour du Mont Blanc, Europe**—This 110-mile trek encircles the Mont Blanc massif, crossing France, Italy, and Switzerland.

5. **Camino de Santiago, Spain**—This is a historic pilgrimage route leading to the cathedral of Santiago de Compostela.

6. **Mount Kilimanjaro, Tanzania** - Africa's highest peak offers several routes to the summit, each promising awe-inspiring vistas.

7. **Everest Base Camp, Nepal** - This trail offers hikers a chance to experience the majestic Himalayas and the culture of the Sherpa people.

8. **The Overland Track, Australia** - A 40-mile journey through Tasmania's stunning wilderness areas.

9. **Milford Track, New Zealand** - Known as "the finest walk in the world," it showcases the breathtaking fjords of Fiordland National Park.

10. **Laugavegur Trail, Iceland** - A trek through otherworldly landscapes of glaciers, hot springs, and volcanic fields.

11. **West Coast Trail, Canada** - A challenging 47-mile hike along Vancouver Island's rugged coastline.

12. **GR20, Corsica, France** - A demanding 112-mile trail across the mountainous terrain of Corsica.

13. **The Great Wall of China, China**—Hiking sections of this ancient wall offer a unique insight into China's history and landscapes.

14. **Tongariro Alpine Crossing, New Zealand** - A day hike across volcanic terrain, offering views of emerald lakes and majestic peaks.

15. **Kungsleden, Sweden**—The "King's Trail" is in the Arctic wilderness of Swedish Lapland. It features pristine landscapes and the chance to see the Northern Lights.

Each trail offers a unique adventure, from cultural pilgrimages to high-altitude treks, showcasing the incredible diversity of our planet's landscapes.

Appalachian Trail, USA

The Appalachian Trail (AT) is one of the world's most iconic long-distance hiking paths, stretching approximately 2,200 miles from Springer Mountain in Georgia to Mount Katahdin in Maine. This colossal trail traverses 14 states, crossing diverse landscapes, including dense forests, serene lakes, and high peaks of the Appalachian Mountains. It's not just the physical challenge that draws thousands of hikers each year but also the profound experience of America's vast natural beauty and the unique sense of community among trail-goers.

The AT offers a variety of experiences, from challenging mountain ascents to leisurely walks through pastoral landscapes. Hikers encounter a rich tapestry of American history, culture, and unparalleled scenic vistas. The trail is punctuated with shelters and towns where hikers can resupply and connect with fellow trekkers. Whether in sections or a single thru-hike, completing the AT is a significant achievement in the hiking community, symbolizing physical endurance and a deep engagement with the natural world. The trail embodies the spirit of adventure and the pursuit of personal challenge, making it a must-do for severe hikers around the globe.

Pacific Crest Trail, USA

The Pacific Crest Trail (PCT) is a monumental journey of 2,650 miles, stretching from the arid borders of Mexico in California to the lush forests of British Columbia, Canada. It traverses three states: California, Oregon, and Washington, showcasing the incredible diversity of the American West's landscapes. From the scorching deserts of the Mojave to the glacier-capped peaks of the Sierra Nevada and Cascade ranges, the PCT offers an unparalleled experience of the natural world.

Hiking the PCT is a formidable challenge that demands physical prowess, mental resilience, and thorough preparation. The trail winds through 25 national forests and seven national parks, presenting hikers with breathtaking views and diverse ecosystems. Hikers are immersed in the stunning beauty of wildflower-covered meadows, deep forests, volcanic peaks, and pristine lakes, each step offering a new perspective on the natural splendor of the western United States.

The PCT is not only a journey through nature but also a journey of self-discovery and community. Many embark on the trail seeking solitude and personal growth, finding a vibrant community of fellow hikers, trail angels, and supportive towns along the way, and completing the PCT, whether in one continuous thru-hike or sections over the years, represents a significant personal achievement and a deep connection to the natural environment.

The trail has captured the imagination of hikers worldwide, further popularized by accounts like Cheryl Strayed's "Wild," highlighting the transformative power of such an epic journey. For those who undertake it, the PCT is more than a trail; it's a pilgrimage through the heart of the American wilderness, offering a unique blend of challenge, adventure, and natural beauty.

Inca Trail, Peru

The Inca Trail to Machu Picchu is not merely a path but a journey back in time, weaving through the heart of the Andes to the ancient ruins of Machu Picchu. This 26-mile trek encapsulates the mystical allure of the Incan civilization, offering a blend of breathtaking natural landscapes, architectural marvels, and a deep dive into centuries-old cultures. The trail starts in the Sacred Valley near Ollantaytambo. It takes hikers through various environments, including cloud forests, alpine tundra, and subtropical jungles, culminating in the iconic Sun Gate view of Machu Picchu at sunrise.

Hiking the Inca Trail is a profound experience that challenges the body and captivates the spirit. The path is strewn with ancient stone steps, ruins, and tunnels, offering hikers a tangible connection to the Incan past. The route's altitude, reaching over 13,000 feet at its highest point, demands acclimatization and physical preparation, making the journey as rewarding as it is demanding.

The Inca Trail's limited access, controlled by a permit system to preserve its integrity, adds to its allure. Only 500 permits are issued daily, including guides and porters, ensuring a more intimate experience of the trail and minimizing environmental impact. This regulation underscores the trail's sacredness and the importance of preservation efforts.

Embarking on the Inca Trail is an immersive experience beyond conventional hiking. It's an opportunity to walk in the footsteps of the Incas, surrounded by the majestic beauty of the Andes and enriched by Peru's cultural heritage. The journey offers introspection and connection with the ancient world, culminating in the awe-inspiring sight of Machu Picchu. It stands as a testament to human ingenuity and the enduring spirit of the Incan people, making it a must-do pilgrimage for adventurers and history enthusiasts alike.

Tour du Mont Blanc, Europe

The Tour du Mont Blanc (TMB) is one of the world's most prestigious long-distance hiking trails, offering an unparalleled trekking experience that circles the Mont Blanc massif. Covering approximately 170 kilometers (over 100 miles) and passing through three countries—France, Italy, and Switzerland—the TMB showcases Europe's alpine splendor. The route affords hikers panoramic views of glaciers, alpine meadows, and crystal-clear lakes, set against the backdrop of some of the highest peaks in the Alps, including the towering Mont Blanc.

Embarking on the TMB is to journey through the heart of European alpine culture and history. The trail weaves through charming villages and towns, allowing trekkers to experience the Savoie region's unique cultural and culinary heritage in France, the Aosta Valley in Italy, and the Valais canton in Switzerland. Each trail segment offers its distinctive flavor, from the rich cheeses and wines to the architectural marvels that dot the landscape.

The TMB is renowned not only for its breathtaking scenery but also for its accessibility to hikers of various skill levels. With well-marked paths and numerous refuges and chalets along the route, hikers can choose between challenging themselves with full-day treks or taking more strolls between accommodations. This flexibility makes the TMB popular for seasoned trekkers seeking a challenging adventure and casual walkers looking for a scenic and culturally rich hiking experience.

Despite its popularity, the TMB requires careful preparation and respect for the mountain environment. The weather in the Alps can change rapidly, presenting hikers with challenges such as steep inclines, snowfields, and high-altitude passes. Proper gear, physical conditioning, and an understanding of mountain safety are essential for a successful trek.

The TMB is not just a hike; it explores the natural beauty and human heritage that have shaped the Alpine region. Completing the Tour du Mont Blanc is an achievement that offers a profound sense of accomplishment and connection to the majesty of the mountains. It stands as a testament to the allure of the Alps and the spirit of adventure that draws hikers from around the globe to undertake this remarkable journey.

Camino de Santiago, Spain

The Camino de Santiago, also known as the Way of Saint James, is not merely a trail but a centuries-old pilgrimage leading to the revered shrine of the apostle Saint James the Great in the Cathedral of Santiago de Compostela in Galicia, Spain. Unlike traditional hikes that may focus purely on physical challenge or natural beauty, the Camino offers a unique blend of spiritual journeying, cultural immersion, and physical trekking across the diverse landscapes of Spain.

Spanning a network of routes, the most famous is the Camino Francés, which stretches about 780 kilometers (nearly 500 miles) from Saint-Jean-Pied-de-Port, France, to Santiago de Compostela. This pilgrimage is rich in history and tradition. The path traverses lush forests, rolling hills, medieval towns, and bustling cities, each with its own stories and monuments, providing a walking tour through time.

The Camino de Santiago attracts thousands of pilgrims, or "peregrinos," from across the globe each year. They are drawn not only by religious devotion but also by the search for personal introspection, community, and a break from the pace of modern life. The symbolic scallop shell marks the way, guiding hikers across varied terrains and offering moments of profound connection—to oneself, to nature, and the fellow pilgrims sharing the path.

Hikers on the Camino can expect to experience a deep sense of camaraderie. Comunal hostels, known as "allergies," provide rest and respite, and shared meals and stories foster a unique bond among travelers. This spirit of community and the simplicity of walking day after day offer a transformative experience, stripping away the complexities of daily life and focusing on the rhythm of steps, breath, and the beauty of the Spanish countryside.

Preparation for the Camino de Santiago involves physical readiness and a mental and spiritual openness to the journey's challenges and rewards. While the physical demands vary across the different routes, with some sections more challenging than others, the Camino is accessible to people of all ages and fitness levels, with many choosing to walk portions of the trail that match their ability.

Completing the Camino de Santiago is often described as a life-changing experience, offering a sense of achievement and new perspectives and insights gained along the way. Whether undertaken as a religious pilgrimage, a cultural adventure, or a personal quest, the Camino de Santiago stands as a testament to the enduring human spirit, inviting all who walk its path to discover not just the heart of Spain but also the depths of their resilience, kindness, and capacity for joy.

Mount Kilimanjaro, Tanzania

Mount Kilimanjaro, the highest peak in Africa, rises majestically above the Tanzanian landscape, offering adventurers from around the world the opportunity to stand atop one of the globe's most iconic summits. At 5,895 meters (19,341 feet) above sea level, Kilimanjaro is Africa's tallest mountain and the world's highest free-standing mountain, a solitary giant that dominates the surrounding savannah. The journey to its summit passes through five distinct ecological zones, from the cultivated lower slopes and lush rainforest to the alpine desert and the icy arctic conditions at the peak, providing a trek as varied in the scenery as it is in a challenge.

Climbing Kilimanjaro is a feat that attracts thousands of hikers annually, drawn not only by the physical challenge but also by the profound beauty and unique biodiversity along its routes. The mountain offers several routes to the summit, including the popular Marangu, Machame, and Lemosho routes, each varying in length, difficulty, and scenery, allowing climbers to choose the path that best suits their experience, ability, and interests.

The ascent of Kilimanjaro is a non-technical climb, making it accessible to determined trekkers without the need for specialized mountaineering skills. However, the high altitude, low temperatures, and potential for acute mountain sickness (AMS) demand careful preparation, acclimatization, and respect for the mountain's challenges. Successful climbers are rewarded not only with the physical triumph of reaching the summit but also with stunning views of the African plains below and the unparalleled sense of accomplishment that comes from standing on the roof of Africa.

Embarking on a Kilimanjaro trek is a journey of self-discovery and endurance, a test of physical and mental resilience. Preparation involves physical conditioning, researching, and planning for the trek's logistical and environmental demands. Climbers are encouraged to go with experienced guides and porters, who provide invaluable support and insight into the mountain's environment, ensuring a safe and enriching experience.

The climb also offers a cultural dimension, as hikers often start and finish their journeys in nearby towns and villages, providing a glimpse into the lives and traditions of the Tanzanian people. The experience of climbing Kilimanjaro extends beyond the mountain itself, encompassing the warmth and hospitality of the local communities and the shared camaraderie among climbers.

Climbing Mount Kilimanjaro is more than just a hike; it is an expedition that tests the limits of human endurance and spirit. It is an opportunity to connect deeply with the natural world, experiencing the awe of the Earth's beauty from one of its most majestic vantage points. For many, the journey leaves an indelible mark, a reminder of the mountain's timeless majesty and the profound personal transformations that can occur when we dare to reach beyond our limits.

Everest Base Camp, Nepal

Trekking to Everest Base Camp in Nepal epitomizes the pinnacle of hiking adventures, attracting trekkers from across the globe to the heart of the Himalayas. Situated at an elevation of 5,364 meters (17,598 feet), the base camp is the launching point for mountaineers aiming to summit Everest, the world's highest peak. For trekkers, reaching the base camp is an achievement that offers breathtaking views of some of the highest mountains on Earth and a profound sense of accomplishment.

The trek typically begins in Lukla, following a flight from Kathmandu into the Tenzing-Hillary Airport, one of the most dramatic airfields in the world. From Lukla, the trail winds through the Khumbu region, home to the Sherpa people, whose culture and hospitality are as integral to the journey as the stunning landscapes. Trekkers pass through verdant valleys, serene monasteries, and traditional villages, with the majestic peaks of the Himalayas towering overhead.

The route to Everest Base Camp is dotted with teahouses and lodges, providing rest and respite for trekkers. The trail offers a challenging but attainable trek for those in good physical condition, with acclimatization days built into itineraries to mitigate the risks of altitude sickness. The trek's highlights include the awe-inspiring vistas from Kala Patthar. This viewpoint offers panoramic views of Everest, Nuptse, and Changtse and the opportunity to stand at the foot of the world's highest mountain.

Reaching Everest Base Camp is a journey through an ever-changing tapestry of landscapes, from the lush vegetation of the lower valleys to the stark, glacier-covered expanses near base camp. It's a trek that challenges the body and elevates the spirit, offering moments of introspection and connection with nature that are as breathtaking as the mountains.

The significance of the trek extends beyond the personal achievement of reaching base camp; it's a pilgrimage through a region steeped in mountaineering history and a testament to Everest's enduring allure. Trekkers leave with a deeper appreciation for the mountain environment, the human spirit's resilience, and the Sherpa community's warmth and strength.

Embarking on the Everest Base Camp trek is to follow in the footsteps of legendary mountaineers and to experience the majesty of the Himalayas in a way that few other journeys can offer. It's an adventure that combines physical challenge, cultural immersion, and the raw beauty of nature, culminating in an unforgettable experience that repeatedly draws trekkers back to Nepal's mountains.

The Overland Track, Australia

The Overland Track is prestigious among the world's great hikes, offering an immersive journey through the heart of Tasmania's pristine wilderness. Spanning approximately 65 kilometers (40 miles) in Tasmania's Cradle Mountain-Lake St Clair National Park, part of the Tasmanian Wilderness World Heritage Area, this trek showcases breathtaking landscapes, from dense rainforests and alpine meadows to towering mountains and tranquil lakes.

Starting at the iconic Cradle Mountain and ending at the stunning Lake St Clair, the Overland Track demands respect and preparation from those who walk it. It typically takes six days to complete. The trail leads adventurers across diverse terrains, each day presenting new wonders: cascading waterfalls, glacial valleys, and ancient rainforests filled with unique flora and fauna. This diversity captivates the senses and offers a profound connection with nature, untouched by modern interference.

The track is renowned for its well-maintained paths, comfortable huts, and clear signage, making it accessible to hikers with moderate experience. Despite these conveniences, the unpredictable Tasmanian weather adds an element of challenge, requiring trekkers to be well-prepared with appropriate gear and clothing. The journey is not just a physical challenge but an opportunity to detach from the fast pace of contemporary life and immerse oneself in the tranquility of the wilderness.

The Overland Track also offers side trips for those wishing to explore beyond the main path, including ascents of Cradle Mountain and Mount Ossa – Tasmania's highest peak. These detours provide even more stunning vistas and opportunities for solitude amidst the raw beauty of Tasmania's landscapes.

Conservation is a vital component of the Overland Track experience. Hikers must book their trip in advance during the primary hiking season, limiting the number of people on the trail at any time to reduce environmental impact. This stewardship ensures that the wilderness remains pristine for future generations, preserving its beauty and biodiversity.

Completing the Overland Track is more than just a physical accomplishment; it's an enriching experience that offers insights into the natural history of Tasmania and the importance of preserving such wild places. Hikers come away with memories of the stunning vistas and challenging treks and a deeper appreciation for the delicate balance of ecosystems and the value of conservation efforts.

The Overland Track is a unique gem that encapsulates the essence of adventure and the quest for harmony with nature. It's a journey that challenges the body, ignites the mind, and rejuvenates the spirit. This makes it a must-do for trekkers drawn to Tasmania's unparalleled beauty and untamed wilderness.

The Milford Track, New Zealand

Revered as "The Finest Walk in the World," the Milford Track in New Zealand is a testament to the awe-inspiring natural beauty of Fiordland National Park. Stretching over 53 kilometers (33 miles) from Lake Te Anau to Milford Sound, this track guides adventurers through the heart of New Zealand's wild and pristine landscapes, offering an unforgettable journey through rainforests, alpine passes, and spectacular waterfalls.

We are embarking on the Milford Track journeys through diverse ecosystems and stunning scenery. The track begins at the head of Lake Te Anau, leading hikers across boardwalks through lush, moss-draped forests. The path winds beside clear streams and rivers, opening up to views of towering mountains and cascading waterfalls, including the majestic Sutherland Falls, one of the world's tallest and most spectacular waterfalls.

One of the trek's highlights is the passage over Mackinnon Pass, the track's highest point, offering panoramic views of the surrounding peaks and valleys carved by glaciers millennia ago. The descent from the pass brings hikers into the serene beauty of the Arthur Valley, leading eventually to the dramatic fjords of Milford Sound, a World Heritage site renowned for its towering cliffs and waterfalls plunging directly into the dark waters of the sound.

The Milford Track is a physical journey and a spiritual experience, inviting hikers to connect with the elemental forces of nature. The track's design and the Department of Conservation's management ensure it remains a sustainable and eco-friendly adventure. Hikers must book their journey in advance, as access is limited to preserve the track's natural beauty and minimize human impact on the fragile ecosystem.

Trekking the Milford Track requires preparation and respect for New Zealand's unpredictable weather—parts of the track cross through areas prone to sudden changes in conditions. Proper gear, including waterproof clothing and sturdy boots, is essential, as is a readiness to embrace the challenges and rewards of backcountry hiking.

The Milford Track experience is enhanced by the camaraderie among hikers and their shared appreciation for the beauty of Fiordland. The journey concludes at Milford Sound, where the sheer cliffs, lush rainforests, and serene sound leave an indelible mark on the hearts of those who witness it. This final vista encapsulates the essence of the Milford Track—a celebration of the natural world's power, beauty, and serenity.

Completing the Milford Track enables hikers to achieve a physical feat and gain a profound appreciation for New Zealand's natural heritage. The journey embodies the spirit of adventure and the deep human connection to the Earth, making it a bucket-list experience for trekkers and nature lovers from around the globe.

The Laugavegur Trail, Iceland

Iceland's Laugavegur Trail is a mesmerizing 55-kilometer (34-mile) trek encapsulating the raw, elemental beauty of the island's otherworldly landscapes. Connecting the Landmannalaugar geothermal area to Þórsmörk (Thorsmork) Valley, the trail offers one of the most unique and visually stunning hiking experiences. For those who venture onto its path, the Laugavegur Trail presents an unforgettable journey through a land of contrasting natural wonders—from steaming volcanic fields and icy glaciers to lush valleys and rainbow-colored mountains.

The trek typically spans four to five days, each day unveiling new marvels. The journey begins in Landmannalaugar, famed for its rhyolite mountains, whose vibrant hues range from pink to green to yellow, shaped by centuries of volcanic activity. Hikers can bathe in natural hot springs before passing through the starkly beautiful landscape. The trail ascends past the lava fields of Laugahraun, through the black deserts of Mýrdalsjökull glacier, and over the green hills of Emstrur, showcasing Iceland's dramatic contrasts.

One of the trail's highlights is the ascent to Hrafntinnusker, where hikers find themselves amidst a surreal terrain of obsidian fields sparkling under the Nordic sun. The descent into the valley of Þórsmörk reveals a lush oasis bordered by glaciers and rugged mountain peaks, offering a striking contrast to the earlier volcanic landscapes.

Crossing rivers, navigating snowfields, and braving Iceland's unpredictable weather, trekkers on the Laugavegur Trail must be well-prepared for various conditions. Despite its challenges, the trail is accessible to most hikers with a moderate fitness level and some backcountry experience. The route is well-marked, and along the way, there are huts and campsites where hikers can rest and shelter from the elements.

The Laugavegur Trail is a physical journey exploring Earth's primordial forces. Hikers are treated to an ever-changing tapestry of landscapes that seem to capture the essence of the planet's creation—geothermal vents spewing steam into the cold air, rivers carving through ancient lava fields, and glaciers grinding slowly over the land. The experience is both humbling and exhilarating, offering a profound connection to the natural world that is increasingly rare in today's fast-paced society.

Embarking on the Laugavegur Trail is to walk through a living showcase of geological activity, where the Earth's power is palpable, and its beauty is overwhelming. It's a trek that challenges the body, stimulates the senses, and refreshes the spirit. For those seeking adventure, wilderness, and a deep engagement with nature, the Laugavegur Trail in Iceland stands as a pinnacle experience, a journey through landscapes that defy imagination and linger in memory long after the hike is completed.

West Coast Trail, Canada

The West Coast Trail, part of Canada's Pacific Rim National Park Reserve on Vancouver Island, British Columbia, is a rugged 75-kilometer (47-mile) trek renowned for its challenging terrain and breathtaking beauty. Initially established in 1907 as a lifesaving trail for shipwreck survivors along the treacherous Graveyard of the Pacific, it has since become a bucket-list hike for adventurers seeking the raw beauty of Canada's wilderness. The trail stretches between Bamfield and Port Renfrew, offering hikers a profound journey through dense coastal rainforests, unspoiled beaches, and cliffs that offer panoramic views of the Pacific Ocean.

Embarking on the West Coast Trail is an immersive experience connecting hikers to nature's power and majesty. The path weaves through ancient cedar and Sitka spruce forests, crosses crystal-clear streams, and navigates sandy and rocky shorelines. Hikers encounter unique challenges, including ladder climbs, cable cars, and log crossings over rivers and ravines, adding to the trail's allure and sense of adventure.

The West Coast Trail is not just a physical challenge; it's an encounter with the area's diverse ecosystems and rich cultural history. The trail passes through the traditional territories of the Pacheedaht, Ditidaht, and Huu-ay-at First Nations, offering hikers the opportunity to learn about these communities' Indigenous history and contemporary life. Moreover, the trail is dotted with historical artifacts that tell the region's maritime heritage story, including shipwrecks and lighthouses.

The beauty of the West Coast Trail lies in its untouched wilderness and the isolation it offers. Hikers can enjoy pristine beaches, watch stunning sunsets over the ocean, and maybe even catch sight of whales, seals, and sea lions offshore. The dense rainforest canopy teems with wildlife, from black bears and cougars to bald eagles and myriad species of birds and amphibians, allowing for unparalleled wildlife viewing opportunities.

Preparing for the West Coast Trail requires careful planning and preparation. The trail's demanding nature and variable coastal weather necessitate high-quality, waterproof gear and sufficient food and supplies. Hikers must be prepared for mud, rain, and potentially challenging tidal conditions that affect river crossings and beach sections. Despite its challenges, the trail is equipped with designated campgrounds, offering both wild camping adventure and the comfort of basic amenities.

Completing the West Coast Trail is rewarding, offering a deep connection to the natural world. It reminds us of the rugged beauty of Canada's Pacific coast and the importance of preserving these wild places for future generations. For those who undertake its journey, the West Coast Trail is more than just a hike; it is an unforgettable experience of discovery, challenge, and the timeless allure of the wilderness.

The Great Wall of China

The Great Wall of China, one of the world's most awe-inspiring historical landmarks, offers a unique hiking experience that stretches beyond physical activity into a profound journey through time. This magnificent structure, built and rebuilt from the 3rd century BC to the 17th century AD, snakes across China's landscape, covering over 21,000 kilometers (13,000 miles) of diverse terrain, including mountains, plateaus, and deserts. While it is impossible to hike the wall's entire length, several sections have been preserved and are accessible for hikers, each offering a different glimpse into China's vast history and natural beauty.

One of the most popular sections for hiking is the area around Beijing, which includes well-preserved parts such as Jinshanling, Mutianyu, and the unrestored Jiankou. These segments showcase the Great Wall's architectural grandeur and strategic importance, with towering watchtowers, imposing battlements, and breathtaking mountain vistas. Hiking the Great Wall in these areas can be strenuous yet rewarding, with steep climbs and descents challenging even seasoned trekkers.

The experience of walking atop the Great Wall is unparalleled. It's not just the physical exertion but the sensation of stepping through centuries of history. Each stone tells a story of ancient empires, Mongol invasions, and the incredible human effort to build and maintain this vast defensive structure. The views from the wall are equally mesmerizing, offering sweeping panoramas of China's diverse landscapes, from lush forests to rugged mountain ranges.

Hiking the Great Wall also offers a unique cultural immersion. The wall passes through various provinces with customs, cuisine, and traditions. Hikers can explore local villages, meet residents, and learn about the wall's impact on their ancestors' lives. This cultural journey enriches the hiking experience, providing a deeper understanding of China's complex history and vibrant contemporary life.

Preparation is critical to a successful hike on the Great Wall. The terrain can be challenging, with uneven steps and steep inclines, especially in the unrestored sections. Adequate water, food, and proper hiking gear are essential, as is respect for the wall's historical significance and the natural environment it traverses. Guided tours are available and recommended for those unfamiliar with the area or seeking deeper historical insights.

The Great Wall of China is more than a monument; it's a testament to human endurance, creativity, and the desire to connect and protect. Hiking the wall offers a once-in-a-lifetime experience beyond the physical to touch the heart of China's heritage. It's an adventure that challenges the body, stimulates the mind, and enriches the soul. It leaves hikers with memories that last a lifetime and a profound respect for this monumental feat of ancient engineering.

Tongariro Alpine Crossing, New Zealand

The Tongariro Alpine Crossing in New Zealand is celebrated as one of the world's greatest single-day treks. It offers an awe-inspiring journey through the heart of the North Island's Tongariro National Park, a UNESCO World Heritage site. Spanning 19.4 kilometers (about 12 miles), this hike traverses a remarkable volcanic landscape that is not only of significant natural beauty but also of cultural importance to the Māori people.

The trek starts at the Mangatepopo Valley, gently ascending through old lava flows under the shadow of Mount Ngauruhoe, famously depicted as Mount Doom in the "Lord of the Rings" films. This stark moonscape terrain quickly captivates hikers with its raw beauty, leading to the South Crater, an expansive, flat area that seems a world away from the lush greenery of much of New Zealand.

The climb to the Red Crater, the highest point of the crossing at 1,886 meters (6,188 feet), presents a challenging ascent but rewards hikers with breathtaking views of the Oturere Valley, Mount Tongariro, and the dramatic, steaming vents of the active volcanic crater. The descent from here is equally stunning, with the Emerald Lakes shimmering in volcanic craters, their brilliant colors starkly contrasting with the surrounding landscape of ash and lava.

Continuing, the path winds past the large, blue expanse of the Blue Lake, sacred to the Māori, and then through tussock-covered slopes down to the Ketetahi Hut. The final stretch of the hike descends through lush forest, filled with the calls of native birds, leading to the Ketetahi car park, the endpoint of this epic journey.

The Tongariro Alpine Crossing is known for its unpredictable weather, ranging from clear, sunny skies to cold, rainy conditions, even in summer. This variability, combined with the challenging terrain, requires thorough preparation. Hikers must equip themselves with plenty of water, food, and layers of clothing to adapt to changing conditions. Despite its challenges, the trek remains accessible to individuals with moderate fitness and determination, with thousands completing the crossing each year.

Beyond its physical demands, the crossing offers a spiritual experience deeply rooted in the Māori culture. The mountains of Tongariro National Park are considered sacred, and hikers are encouraged to respect the land by adhering to the principles of "Leave No Trace" and recognizing the spiritual significance of the places they traverse.

The Tongariro Alpine Crossing is more than a hike; it's an adventure that immerses you in the powerful forces of nature, the rich tapestry of Māori culture, and the breathtaking beauty of New Zealand's wilderness. It's a journey that challenges the body, engages the senses, and enriches the spirit, leaving an indelible mark on all who undertake it.

The Kungsleden, Sweden

The Kungsleden, or "The King's Trail," is Sweden's premier long-distance trek and one of the most famous hiking trails in the world. Stretching approximately 440 kilometers (about 270 miles) through the Swedish Lapland, it traverses one of Europe's last significant wilderness areas, offering an unparalleled adventure into the Arctic landscape. The trail, established in the early 20th century by the Swedish Tourist Association, begins in Abisko in the north and extends south to Hemavan, taking hikers through the vast, untouched beauty of the Scandinavian mountains.

The Kungsleden passes through four national parks: Abisko, Stora Sjöfallet, Sarek, and Padjelanta, each offering unique landscapes and natural wonders. From the majestic alpine world of Abisko, known for its clear blue lakes and dramatic mountain vistas, to the rich biodiversity and deep forests of Sarek, the trail offers diverse experiences. Hikers can marvel at the sight of Sweden's highest peak, Kebnekaise, explore the Laponia area—a UNESCO World Heritage site—or relax beside the tranquil waters of Lake Tärnasjön.

The journey on the Kungsleden is marked by well-maintained paths and bridges, with strategically placed huts and cabins along the route, providing shelter and basic amenities. This accessibility makes the trail suitable for seasoned trekkers and those new to long-distance hiking. The trail is traditionally divided into sections, allowing hikers to tackle the trek in smaller, manageable parts, with the most popular segment being the northernmost 110 kilometers (68 miles) from Abisko to Nikkaluokta.

Hiking the Kungsleden is to experience the sublime beauty of the Arctic wilderness—the silence of its vast expanses, the purity of its air, and the ever-changing light that dances across the landscape. The summer brings the midnight sun, with almost 24 hours of daylight, while late summer and early fall paint the terrain in brilliant colors. Hikers might encounter reindeer herds, witness the aurora borealis, and enjoy the rich flora and fauna of the region.

Preparation is vital for those embarking on the Kungsleden. The weather can be unpredictable, with conditions ranging from sunny and warm to cold and rainy, even in summer. Proper gear, including warm clothing, rain protection, and sturdy hiking boots, is essential. Additionally, hikers should be prepared for the physical demands of the trail, though the ability to choose segments of the hike allows for a customized trekking experience.

The Kungsleden is more than just a trail; it's a journey into the heart of the Arctic wilderness. It offers a chance to disconnect from the modern world and connect with nature in its most primal form. For those seeking solitude, adventure, and the raw beauty of the natural world, the Kungsleden is a trek that promises to be an unforgettable experience, offering a deeper understanding of the landscape, the wildlife, and the enduring appeal of the great outdoors.

Exploring the wilderness through hiking nurtures our connection to nature and challenges our physical and mental limits. As hikers progress in their adventures, they often seek out more challenging and rugged terrains requiring advanced hiking techniques. Mastering these techniques enhances safety, increases efficiency, and amplifies the enjoyment of exploring remote landscapes.

Adapting to Varied Terrain

Advanced hiking often involves traversing diverse terrains, each presenting unique challenges requiring specific skills for safe and effective navigation.

Rocky and Uneven Terrain

- **Technique:** Focus on maintaining a low center of gravity to enhance balance. Use a "three points of contact" approach when climbing or descending steep sections, ensuring stability at all times.

- **Gear Tip:** Wear boots with good ankle support and a sole with excellent grip. Trekking poles can significantly improve balance.

River Crossings

- **Technique:** Assess the river's speed and depth before crossing. Use trekking poles for additional support, and face upstream when crossing fast-flowing sections to maintain balance.

- **Safety Tip:** Unbuckle your backpack before crossing to ensure you can easily remove it if you fall into the water.

Snow and Ice

- **Technique:** Learn to use crampons and an ice axe for stability and safety on icy terrain. Practice self-arrest techniques with the ice axe to stop yourself if you slip and start sliding.

- **Preparation:** Understand the signs of avalanche danger and take an avalanche safety course if you plan on hiking in avalanche-prone areas during winter or spring.

Advanced Navigation Skills

Beyond basic map and compass skills, advanced hikers must be proficient in navigating challenging landscapes where trails may not be well-marked, or GPS signals are unreliable.

Topographic Map Mastery

- **Skill Development:** Learn to read and interpret topographic maps accurately, including understanding contour lines, identifying key terrain features, and estimating elevations and distances.

- **Application:** Use your topographic map skills to navigate off-trail or in complex terrain, planning your route based on the landscape's physical features.

GPS and Tech Navigation

- **Utilization:** Besides traditional navigation tools, become proficient with GPS devices and smartphone navigation apps that offer offline maps and satellite imagery.

- **Backup Plan:** Always carry a physical map and compass as a backup, and ensure your devices have sufficient battery power.

Endurance and Conditioning

Long-distance and challenging hikes require excellent physical conditioning and endurance to prevent injuries and ensure an enjoyable experience.

Cardiovascular Fitness

- **Training:** Incorporate regular cardiovascular exercises, such as running, cycling, or swimming, into your routine to improve heart and lung efficiency.

- **Practice Hikes:** Use practice hikes that mimic your planned hikes' distance and elevation gain to condition your body and identify areas needing improvement.

Strength and Flexibility

- **Routine:** Develop a strength-training routine focusing on the legs, core, and upper body to support the demands of carrying a backpack and navigating rugged terrain.

- **Flexibility:** Incorporate stretching or yoga into your fitness regimen to improve flexibility, reduce the risk of muscle strains, and enhance recovery.

Mental Preparedness

Advanced hiking tests physical capabilities and mental resilience. Being mentally prepared for the challenges ahead is crucial for a successful hike.

Adaptability

- **Mindset:** Cultivate a flexible mindset that can adapt to changing conditions, unexpected challenges, and the need to alter plans for safety reasons.

- **Stress Management:** Develop techniques such as deep breathing or positive visualization to maintain calm and focus during difficult situations.

Risk Assessment and Decision-Making

- **Skills:** Enhance your ability to assess risks accurately and make informed decisions quickly, whether related to weather conditions, terrain challenges, or potential hazards.

- **Knowledge:** Continuously educate yourself about the environments you plan to hike in, including local wildlife, weather patterns, and everyday hazards.

Advancing your hiking skills opens the door to exploring some of the most breathtaking and remote areas of the natural world. You can confidently embark on more ambitious hikes by mastering advanced techniques for varied terrain, honing navigation skills, conditioning your body for endurance, and preparing mentally for the challenges ahead. These skills ensure your safety and enjoyment on the trail and deepen your connection to the wilderness, encouraging a lifelong pursuit of adventure and exploration.

Embarking on hiking adventures introduces enthusiasts to various terrains, each with unique challenges and rewards. Mastery of specific hiking techniques tailored to different terrains enhances trail safety, efficiency, and enjoyment.

Forest and Woodland Terrain

Hiking through dense forests and woodlands offers a serene experience, with trails often cushioned by layers of leaf litter or pine needles. However, the uneven ground, roots, and potentially slippery conditions demand cautious navigation.

Technique Focus:

- **Watch Your Step:** Look at the trail ahead for roots, rocks, and uneven ground that could cause trips or twisted ankles.

- **Pace Yourself:** Dense tree cover can make judging the time of day and distance covered harder. Maintain a steady pace and take regular breaks to avoid exhaustion.

- **Trail Etiquette:** Stick to marked trails to protect undergrowth and habitat. Yield to uphill hikers and share the trail respectfully with all users.

Mountain and Alpine Terrain

Mountainous and alpine terrains present some of the most physically demanding and visually rewarding hiking experiences. These environments require careful planning and acute awareness of the weather and potential altitude effects.

Technique Focus:

- **Acclimatization:** Take time to acclimatize to higher altitudes to avoid altitude sickness. This may mean planning a gradual ascent over several days.

- **Use of Trekking Poles:** Trekking poles can significantly reduce the impact on knees during descents and provide additional stability on uneven terrain.

- **Layer Clothing:** Temperatures can vary dramatically in mountainous terrain. Wear layers that can be easily added or removed to manage body temperature.

Desert Terrain

Hiking in desert terrain offers an encounter with stark beauty and extreme conditions. Preparation is critical to managing the heat, scarce water sources, and challenging navigation across vast, featureless landscapes.

Technique Focus:

- **Hydration:** Carry more water than you think you'll need and plan your route around water sources. Avoid hiking during the peak heat of the day.

- **Sun Protection:** Wear a wide-brimmed hat, sunglasses, and long sleeves to protect against sun exposure. Apply sunscreen regularly.

- **Navigation Skills:** Deserts often lack distinct landmarks. Be proficient with a GPS device and understand how to use a compass and map for navigation.

Snow and Ice Terrain

Hiking in snow and ice-covered landscapes requires specialized equipment and skills to safely navigate slippery and treacherous paths.

Technique Focus:

- **Crampons and Ice Axes:** Learn how to use crampons for traction on ice and snow properly, and practice using an ice axe for stability and self-arrest techniques.

- **Layer for Warmth:** Dress in moisture-wicking base and insulating layers, and carry a waterproof outer layer to protect from wet conditions.

- **Avalanche Safety:** Understand avalanche risks, learn to recognize hazardous conditions, and carry appropriate avalanche safety gear when hiking in prone areas.

Coastal and Beach Terrain

Coastal hikes can be deceivingly challenging, with soft sand for strenuous walking and exposure to elements like wind and salt spray.

Technique Focus:

- **Footwear:** Choose closed-toe shoes that offer protection and are comfortable on sand. Be aware that sand can quickly cause blisters.

- **Tide Planning:** Check tide tables to avoid being caught by high tides, especially when routes may be impassable at certain times.

- **Wind Exposure:** Prepare for the lack of shelter from the wind by wearing appropriate clothing and carrying lightweight windbreakers.

Mixed Terrain

Many hiking trails traverse various terrains, presenting various challenges within a single hike. It is crucial to be prepared for changing conditions and adaptable to techniques.

Technique Focus:

- **Flexible Planning:** Be ready to adjust your hiking pace, breaks, and even your route based on the conditions of each terrain type encountered.

- **Gear Adaptability:** Carry a small, versatile pack with gear essentials that can quickly be adjusted for different terrains, such as extra layers or traction devices for your footwear.

- **Continuous Learning:** Each type of terrain offers unique challenges and lessons. Take every hike to learn and improve your skills and techniques.

Navigating diverse terrains requires proper preparation, the right gear, and a keen awareness of your surroundings. Each environment—the dense canopy of forest trails, the rugged slopes of mountain paths, the expansive vistas of desert landscapes, the icy expanse of snow-covered trails, or the scenic routes along coastal areas—offers unique challenges and rewards. By mastering the specific hiking techniques for different terrains, hikers can ensure their safety, increase their efficiency on the trail, and enhance their enjoyment of exploring the natural world. This knowledge empowers hikers to confidently tackle a broader range of landscapes, enriching their outdoor adventures with diverse experiences and deeper connections to the environment.

Exploring the wilderness doesn't have to end when the sun sets or when the warmth of summer fades into the cold embrace of winter. Night and winter hiking present unique challenges but offer equally unique rewards: the tranquility of a landscape bathed in moonlight or the silent, pristine beauty of a snow-covered trail. However, these forms of hiking require additional preparation, gear, and awareness to ensure safety and enjoyment.

Night Hiking Tips

Night hiking can transform a familiar trail into a new world, illuminated by starlight and the glow of your headlamp. The sounds of the forest at night, the cooler temperatures, and the experience of seeing nocturnal wildlife add to the adventure's allure. However, the darkness also complicates navigation and increases the potential for hazards.

Gear Essentials

- **Headlamp and Backup Light:** A reliable headlamp, which offers hands-free illumination, is one of your most crucial pieces of equipment. Always carry extra batteries or a backup light source.

- **Reflective Gear:** Wear clothing or a backpack with reflective patches to increase visibility, especially if your trail crosses roads or is shared with cyclists.

Navigation

- **Familiarize with the Trail:** Ideally, hike routes you know well or have hiked during the day. This familiarity helps with navigation when landmarks are more challenging to identify.

- **Map and Compass:** GPS devices are helpful, but always carry a physical map and compass as backups. Practice using them in low-light conditions.

Safety Precautions

- **Inform Someone:** Always let someone know your plan, including your route and expected return time.

- **Buddy System:** Hike with a partner or group for added safety. If you must hike alone, be extra cautious and stay on well-known, less challenging trails.

- **Wildlife Awareness:** Understand the nocturnal animals you might encounter and how to observe or avoid them safely.

Winter Hiking Tips

Winter transforms the hiking landscape, offering breathtaking views of snow-covered trees and frozen lakes. However, it also brings significant challenges, including colder temperatures, shorter days, and the potential for snow and ice on the trail.

Gear Essentials

- **Layered Clothing:** Dress in layers to manage body heat and moisture. Include a moisture-wicking base layer, an insulating layer, and a waterproof outer layer.

- **Winter Hiking Boots:** Insulated, waterproof boots are essential for keeping your feet warm and dry. Pair them with wool or synthetic socks.

- **Traction Devices:** Snow and ice on the trail require crampons or microspikes for added grip. In deeper snow, snowshoes might be necessary.

Navigation and Trail Conditions

- **Shorter Days:** Plan for shorter hikes to ensure you can return before dark, considering the limited daylight hours.

- **Trail Markers:** Snow can obscure trail markers. Use GPS or a map and compass to navigate, and be prepared to turn back if the trail becomes too difficult to follow.

Cold-Weather Risks

- **Hypothermia Prevention:** Keep dry and avoid sweating. Wet clothing loses its insulating properties and increases the risk of hypothermia.

- **Frostbite Awareness:** Protect extremities, such as fingers, toes, ears, and nose, which are most susceptible to frostbite. Recognize the early signs, including numbness and pale skin, and take immediate action to warm up.

Winter Hiking Strategies

- **Start Early:** Maximize daylight hours by starting your hike early.

- **Pace and Energy:** Cold weather and snow can make hiking more physically demanding. Maintain a steady pace and consume high-energy snacks to keep your energy levels up.

- **Hydration:** It's easy to underestimate how much water you need in cold weather. Use insulated water bottles to prevent freezing, and drink regularly.

Combining Night and Winter Hiking

Hiking at night in winter conditions combines the challenges of both activities. Preparation and caution are paramount. Ensure your headlamp and backup light can operate in cold temperatures, and consider the increased difficulty of navigating snow-covered trails in the dark. Group hikes are remarkably advisable in these conditions for safety and shared experience.

Night and winter hiking offer enriching experiences that connect adventurers with the natural world in profound and unique ways. However, these forms of hiking demand respect for the elements and thorough preparation. By equipping yourself with the right gear, enhancing your navigation skills, understanding the risks, and following safety precautions, you can embrace the beauty and tranquility of the trails under the moonlight or amidst the snowflakes. These tips serve as a foundation for venturing safely into the night and the cold, allowing you to explore the wilderness with confidence and wonder.

Solo Hiking

Solo hiking invites adventurers into a profoundly personal experience with the natural world, offering unparalleled freedom, introspection, and a unique sense of achievement.

Freedom and Flexibility: One of the most significant advantages of solo hiking is complete control over your itinerary. You set the pace, choose the trail, and decide when to take breaks, allowing a custom-fit adventure aligned with your desires and physical capabilities.

Self-Reliance and Skills Development: Hiking alone demands a high level of self-reliance. You are solely responsible for navigating, setting up camp, and dealing with challenges. This environment fosters rapid growth in outdoor skills and confidence in one's abilities to manage in the wilderness.

Solitude and Introspection: Solo hiking provides a rare opportunity for solitude, offering a space for meditation and reflection free from the distractions of everyday life. The tranquility of nature can facilitate profound personal insights and a deeper connection to the environment.

Considerations and Precautions:

- **Safety:** The biggest concern with solo hiking is safety. Without companions to assist in an emergency, solo hikers must take extra precautions. This includes informing someone about their itinerary, carrying a fully charged phone or a satellite communicator, and being prepared with a well-stocked first aid kit.

- **Loneliness:** For some, the solitude of solo hiking can lead to feelings of loneliness, especially on longer treks. Vital mental preparation and strategies for coping with being alone for extended periods are essential.

Group Hiking

Group hiking brings together individuals with a shared interest in exploring the outdoors, offering social interaction, shared responsibilities, and enhanced safety.

Social Interaction and Camaraderie: One of the joys of group hiking is the companionship it offers. Sharing the trail with others can lead to lasting friendships, enriching conversations, and a supportive atmosphere that enhances the overall experience.

Shared Responsibilities: In a group, tasks such as navigation, cooking, and setting up camp can be distributed among members, lightening the load for everyone. This collaboration can make the logistics of a hiking trip more manageable and enjoyable.

Enhanced Safety: Hiking with others increases safety on the trail. In case of injury or illness, group members can provide immediate assistance and help to evacuate if necessary. There is also safety in numbers when it comes to encountering wildlife.

Considerations and Precautions:

- **Pace and Flexibility:** One challenge of group hiking is managing different fitness levels and hiking preferences. The group must find a pace accommodating all members, which may require compromises on distance covered and trail choice.

- **Group Dynamics:** Group dynamics can influence a group hike's success. Conflicting personalities or differing goals can lead to tension. Clear communication and mutual respect are crucial for maintaining harmony.

Making the Choice

When deciding between solo and group hiking, consider your personal goals for the trip, your experience level, and how you handle solitude versus social settings.

Personal Goals: Are you seeking a profound personal challenge, or are you looking to share the joys of nature with others? Your primary objectives can guide your decision.

Experience Level: Less experienced hikers might benefit from the safety and shared knowledge of a group hike, while seasoned hikers may seek the challenges and rewards of going solo.

Solitude vs. Social Interaction: Reflect on your preference for solitude or social interaction. Some thrive on the quiet reflection of solo hiking, while others prefer the camaraderie and shared experience of hiking with a group.

Both solo and group hiking offer unique opportunities to connect with nature and oneself. Solo hiking provides freedom, challenges personal limits, and offers solitude for introspection. In contrast, group hiking offers shared experiences, the safety of companionship, and the joy of exploring the wilderness with others. Ultimately, the choice between solo and group hiking depends on personal preferences, goals, and the specific circumstances of each trip. Whichever you choose, the trails offer endless adventures and insights waiting to be discovered by those willing to step forward into the journey.

Integrating technology into hiking represents a paradigm shift in how adventurers interact with the natural world. From navigation aids to fitness tracking and environmental conservation efforts, technology has enhanced the hiking experience, making it safer, more accessible, and more engaging for a broader audience. This exploration delves into the multifaceted relationship between technology and hiking, examining its benefits, considerations, and the future of this integration.

Enhancing Navigation and Safety

GPS devices and smartphone apps have revolutionized trail navigation, reducing the likelihood of getting lost and increasing safety for hikers of all experience levels.

GPS Devices and Smartphone Apps: Devices like handheld GPS and smartphones equipped with apps such as AllTrails, Gaia GPS, and ViewRanger offer detailed maps, trail data, and real-time location tracking. This technology allows hikers to navigate confidently, even on remote or poorly marked trails.

Emergency Communication: Satellite messengers and Personal Locator Beacons (PLBs) provide a lifeline in emergencies, enabling hikers to send distress signals and location data to rescue services, regardless of cell coverage.

Considerations: While technology has made navigation and safety more manageable, relying on something other than electronic devices is crucial. Battery failure or damage can render devices useless. Therefore, carrying a traditional map and compass and knowing how to use them remains essential.

Promoting Fitness and Health

Technology has also significantly influenced hikers' achievement of fitness goals, providing tools to track progress, set challenges, and share achievements.

Fitness Trackers and Smartwatches: Devices like Fitbit, Garmin, and Apple Watch track physical activity, monitor heart rate, and estimate calories burned, allowing hikers to set and monitor fitness goals. Integration with apps can create a social aspect of hiking, encouraging users through shared challenges and achievements.

Training Apps: Apps designed for hiking preparation offer structured training plans, tips, and exercises to improve fitness levels and help hikers tackle more challenging treks.

Considerations: While fitness trackers and apps can motivate and improve health, listening to your body and not pushing beyond safe limits is essential. Technology should supplement, not dictate, physical activity levels.

Enhancing the Hiking Experience

Technology not only aids in navigation and fitness but also enriches the hiking experience by providing access to a wealth of information and enabling the sharing of adventures.

Educational Apps: Apps that offer information on flora, fauna, geology, and history can enrich the hiking experience, turning a simple walk into an educational journey.

Photography and Social Sharing: Advances in smartphone cameras and portable photography gear have enabled hikers to capture and share their experiences like never before, inspiring others and building communities of outdoor enthusiasts.

Considerations: While documenting hikes can enhance the experience, it's essential to remain present and respectful of nature. Overusing devices can detract from the immersive experience of hiking, and social sharing should be done responsibly to avoid overcrowding and impact sensitive environments.

Conservation and Environmental Awareness

Technology is crucial in conservation efforts. It provides tools for monitoring environmental changes, promotes responsible hiking practices, and fosters a global community of conservation-minded individuals.

Trail and Habitat Monitoring: Drones and remote sensing technology enable conservationists to monitor trails, wildlife, and habitat health, helping to manage access and protect sensitive areas.

Digital Leave No Trace Education: Websites, apps, and social media platforms offer ways to educate hikers on Leave No Trace principles and environmental stewardship, promoting a culture of responsible outdoor activity.

Citizen Science Projects: Apps like iNaturalist encourage hikers to contribute to scientific data collection by documenting wildlife and plant sightings, aiding in biodiversity research and conservation efforts.

Considerations: While technology can aid conservation, it's vital to use it responsibly. Drone usage, for example, is restricted in many areas to prevent wildlife disturbance and privacy breaches.

The Future of Technology and Hiking

As technology continues to evolve, its integration into hiking will likely grow, offering new ways to explore, understand, and protect the natural world. Innovations in wearable tech, augmented reality (AR), and environmental monitoring promise to further enhance and personalize the hiking experience while fostering a deeper connection with nature.

Considerations for the Future: The challenge lies in balancing the benefits of technology with the essence of hiking—disconnecting from the digital world and immersing oneself in the natural environment. Future developments should focus on enhancing safety, education, and conservation while encouraging hikers to engage fully with the outdoor experience.

Technology has undeniably transformed hiking, making it more accessible, safer, and engaging. Technology offers many benefits, from advanced navigation tools and fitness tracking to conservation efforts and community building. However, it's essential to use these tools responsibly, balancing the convenience and insights they provide with the fundamental goal of hiking: to connect with nature. As we look to the future, the thoughtful integration of technology promises to continue enriching the hiking experience, fostering a deeper appreciation for the natural world and motivating a new generation of hikers to explore responsibly.

Harnessing the Power of Navigation Apps

Smartphone navigation apps have become indispensable tools for hikers. They offer detailed maps, trail information, and real-time GPS tracking without a cell signal. These apps provide the convenience of a lightweight, multifunctional device and offer features like trail reviews, difficulty ratings, and user experiences that can aid in planning and executing hikes.

AllTrails and Gaia GPS: Leading apps like AllTrails and Gaia GPS provide extensive libraries of trail maps. They allow users to download maps for offline use, record their hikes, and even share their experiences with a community of fellow hikers. These apps often include safety features, such as location sharing with loved ones, adding an extra layer of security to solo adventures.

Emerging Features: Augmented reality (AR) features are beginning to emerge in navigation apps, offering hikers real-time information overlaid on their physical surroundings. By pointing their smartphone camera at the landscape, users can identify peaks, landmarks, and trail directions, enriching the hiking experience with interactive, educational content.

The Role of Wearable Tech in Hiking

Wearable technology, including smartwatches and fitness trackers, has become a game-changer for hikers seeking to monitor their physical activity and easily navigate. These devices track steps, elevation gain, and heart rate and offer GPS navigation, weather alerts, and emergency features.

Garmin and Suunto: Brands like Garmin and Suunto have developed rugged, outdoor-focused smartwatches that provide detailed topographic maps, breadcrumb trail navigation, and barometric altimeter data, making them powerful tools for wilderness exploration. Their extended battery life and durability in extreme conditions make them reliable companions on the trail.

Safety Features: Advanced safety features, such as SOS alerts and fall detection, can notify emergency contacts or search and rescue teams of the wearer's location, offering peace of mind for both hikers and their families.

Drones: A New Perspective on Hiking Trails

Drones have introduced a novel way of experiencing and documenting hiking trails, offering aerial perspectives that were once only accessible to professional filmmakers. Drones with high-resolution cameras can capture breathtaking landscapes, scout trails, and even assist in search and rescue operations.

Regulations and Considerations: While drones open up new possibilities for exploration and photography, their use is regulated in many protected areas to prevent disturbances to wildlife and other hikers. Hikers must familiarize themselves with local regulations and practice responsible drone flying, prioritizing the preservation of natural environments and the privacy of others.

The Future of Navigation and Tracking Technologies

Emerging technologies continue to push the boundaries of what's possible in outdoor navigation and tracking. Developments in satellite communication, solar charging, and lightweight materials promise to bring even more sophisticated tools to hikers, enhancing safety and convenience on the trail.

Satellite Communication Devices: Devices that enable two-way communication via satellite, such as Garmin's inReach, provide a lifeline in areas without cell coverage, allowing hikers to send and receive messages, share their location, and access weather forecasts.

Solar-Powered Gadgets: Innovations in solar-powered technology offer the potential for devices that can be charged on the go, ensuring that hikers have access to power for their navigation tools and emergency devices, even on multi-day treks in remote areas.

Wearable Tech Innovations: The future of wearable technology promises even more integrated features, including advanced biometric tracking, environmental sensors that monitor air quality and UV exposure, and materials that adapt to temperature changes, providing optimal comfort and safety for hikers.

Integrating apps, gadgets, and emerging technologies into hiking has opened up new horizons for adventurers, offering tools that enhance navigation, improve safety, and enrich the outdoor experience. As these technologies evolve, they promise to make wilderness exploration more accessible and enjoyable, encouraging more people to connect with the natural world. However, it's essential to balance the use of technology with respect for nature and a commitment to preserving the wild places we cherish. By utilizing these tools responsibly and ethically, hikers can enjoy the best of both worlds: the timeless allure of the trail and the benefits of modern innovation.

Photography on the hiking trail is an exquisite blend of art and science, requiring creative vision and technical skill to capture the essence of the wilderness. As hikers traverse through varied landscapes, from majestic mountains to serene forests, photography becomes a way to preserve these moments, share experiences, and express the profound beauty of the natural world. This exploration delves into the art and science of trail photography, offering insights into capturing compelling images that resonate with both the photographer and their audience.

Understanding the Landscape

The foundation of trail photography lies in understanding and connecting with the landscape. Each environment presents its unique characteristics, challenges, and moments of beauty.

Observation and Patience: Successful trail photography often requires patience and observation, waiting for the right light, weather, or moment that captures the essence of the place. It's about seeing beyond the obvious, finding beauty in details often overlooked, and allowing the landscape to reveal its stories.

Composition and Perspective: Composition is crucial in landscape photography. It involves arranging elements within the frame to be aesthetically pleasing and convey the intended message or emotion. Exploring different perspectives—such as shooting from a high vantage point or getting close to the ground—can dramatically change the image's impact, offering fresh interpretations of familiar scenes.

The Science of Light

Light plays a pivotal role in photography, influencing mood, texture, and color. Understanding and harnessing light is essential to creating compelling images.

Golden Hour: The hours shortly after sunrise and before sunset, known as the golden hour, offer soft, warm light that enhances textures and colors, ideal for landscape photography. Planning hikes to coincide with these times can result in stunningly lit scenes.

Weather and Atmospheric Conditions: Overcast days provide diffused light that minimizes shadows and highlights, perfect for capturing the subtleties of color and texture. Mist, fog, and clouds add atmosphere and depth to landscapes, offering opportunities for moody and evocative images.

Technical Mastery

The science of photography also involves mastering the technical aspects of the camera and post-processing techniques to realize the photographer's vision.

Camera Settings: Understanding exposure—aperture, shutter speed, and ISO—is fundamental to controlling how light is captured. Aperture affects depth of field, shutter speed can freeze or blur motion, and ISO impacts image noise, each playing a role in the image's final look.

Lens Choices: Different lenses offer various perspectives. Wide-angle lenses are ideal for capturing expansive landscapes, while telephoto lenses can isolate distant details or compress elements within the scene.

Post-Processing: Digital editing allows photographers to refine their images, adjusting exposure, contrast, and color to match their vision. While post-processing is a powerful tool, the goal is to enhance the scene's natural beauty, not overly alter it.

Ethical Considerations and Conservation

Photography on the hiking trail is responsible for respecting the environment and promoting conservation through ethical practices.

Leave No Trace: Adhering to Leave No Trace principles ensures that photography does not harm the landscape. This includes staying on trails, avoiding sensitive areas, and not disturbing wildlife.

Conservation Awareness: Trail photography can play a significant role in conservation efforts, raising awareness of natural beauty and the importance of protecting these areas. Photographs can inspire others to appreciate and advocate for the environment.

Cultural Sensitivity: When photographing in areas with cultural significance or local communities, it's essential to approach with respect and sensitivity, seeking permission where necessary and being mindful of the impact of your actions.

Sharing Your Vision

The final step in the art and science of trail photography is sharing your work and connecting with others who share your passion for the wilderness.

Social Media and Online Platforms: Platforms like Instagram, 500px, and Flickr offer opportunities to share images, engage with a community of outdoor photographers, and receive feedback.

Photography Exhibits and Publications: Exhibiting your work in galleries or submitting to outdoor magazines and websites can reach a wider audience, allowing your images to inspire and evoke a deeper appreciation for the natural world.

The art and science of photography on the hiking trail are about much more than capturing images; it's a way to engage deeply with the environment, to see the world with fresh eyes, and to share the beauty of the wilderness with others. It combines technical skill with creative vision, challenging photographers to learn and grow continuously. Through ethical and mindful photography, hikers can document their adventures and contribute to appreciating and conservating the natural landscapes they love. In this way, trail photography becomes a powerful medium for storytelling, exploration, and advocacy, capturing moments that speak to the heart of the wilderness experience.

Social media has significantly transformed hiking culture over the last decade, shaping how experiences are shared, trails are discovered, and communities are formed. This digital revolution has brought the once-niche hobby of hiking into the mainstream, offering positive enhancements and challenges to the outdoor community. This exploration delves into the multifaceted role of social media in hiking culture, examining its impact on trail popularity, conservation efforts, community building, and the authenticity of outdoor experiences.

Amplifying Trail Popularity

Social media platforms have become powerful tools for sharing the allure of hidden gems and iconic trails alike. Stunning photographs and engaging stories inspire users to seek new adventures, contributing to an increased interest in hiking and outdoor recreation.

Pros:

- **Accessibility:** Social media democratizes access to information about hiking, making it easier for beginners to find trails that match their skill level and interests.

- **Inspiration:** For many, social media serves as a source of inspiration, showcasing the beauty of nature and encouraging a deeper appreciation for the outdoors.

Cons:

- **Overcrowding:** Popular trails can become overrun, leading to environmental degradation, trail erosion, and a diminished hiking experience for those seeking solitude.

- **Unsafe Behavior:** The desire for social media recognition can lead some to take unnecessary risks, posing safety hazards and potentially requiring rescue operations.

Fostering Community and Inclusion

Social media has played a crucial role in building communities among hikers, connecting individuals who share a passion for the outdoors regardless of geographical boundaries.

Pros:

- **Support and Advice:** Online communities offer a platform for sharing advice, gear recommendations, and trail tips, supporting novice and experienced hikers.

- **Inclusivity:** Social media initiatives and groups focused on outdoor diversity have helped make hiking more inclusive, encouraging participation from underrepresented groups.

Cons:

- **Erosion of Solitude:** As hiking gains popularity through social media, the quest for solitude and a deep connection with nature can become more challenging.

- **Comparison Culture:** Social media can foster a sense of competition or inadequacy, where the value of a hike is judged by the likes or comments it garners rather than the personal experience.

Impact on Conservation and Responsible Hiking

The widespread reach of social media offers an unparalleled opportunity to educate hikers on responsible practices and conservation efforts, though it also poses challenges to environmental stewardship.

Pros:

- **Awareness and Advocacy:** Social media campaigns can raise awareness about conservation issues, mobilize support for protected areas, and promote responsible hiking practices.

- **Citizen Science:** Platforms encouraging sharing flora and fauna observations can contribute valuable data to conservation research and biodiversity monitoring.

Cons:

- **Habitat Disturbance:** The influx of hikers drawn by social media fame can lead to habitat disturbance, wildlife displacement, and damage to sensitive ecosystems.

- **Location Tagging:** Geotagging can concentrate foot traffic to specific locations, exacerbating environmental impacts and altering the natural landscape.

The Authenticity of Outdoor Experiences

As social media becomes increasingly intertwined with hiking culture, it prompts reflection on the authenticity and motivation behind outdoor adventures.

Pros:

- **Personal Narratives:** Social media allows individuals to share their unique hiking experiences, stories of personal growth, and moments of connection with nature, enriching the collective narrative of outdoor culture.

- **Creative Expression:** For many, capturing and sharing photographs or videos of their hikes is a form of creative expression, adding depth to their outdoor experience.

Cons:

- **Performative Hiking:** There's a risk that the pressure to share compelling content on social media can lead to performative hiking, where the experience is tailored for an online audience rather than personal fulfillment.

- **Disconnect from Nature:** The constant focus on documenting and sharing experiences can detract from the immersive and reflective aspects of hiking, potentially diminishing the personal connection with the natural world.

Social media's role in hiking culture is complex and multifaceted, offering opportunities and challenges to the outdoor community. Its influence on trail popularity, community building, conservation efforts, and the authenticity of outdoor experiences underscores the need for a balanced approach to integrating the digital and natural worlds. By promoting responsible social media practices—such as mindful sharing, emphasizing safety, and advocating for conservation—hikers can leverage these platforms to enhance, rather than detract from, the richness of the hiking experience. As we navigate the intersections of technology and nature, it's crucial to remember the core values of hiking: respect for the environment, a sense of adventure, and the pursuit of personal growth and connection with the natural world.

Building a hiking community is more than just sharing trails and tips; it's about fostering a culture of inclusivity, support, and a collective passion for exploring the natural world. Such communities offer a space for individuals to connect over shared experiences, learn from one another, and collectively advocate conserving natural spaces. This exploration delves into the significance of hiking communities, the strategies for building and nurturing them, and the impact they can have on individuals and the broader outdoor culture.

The Foundation of Hiking Communities

At their core, hiking communities are built on a shared love for the outdoors and a mutual respect for the natural environment. They serve as platforms for exchange, where stories, knowledge, and resources can be shared to enhance the hiking experience for all members.

Shared Experiences: Hiking communities thrive on their members' collective experiences. From exhilarating summit successes to challenging weather conditions, shared stories foster a sense of belonging and camaraderie.

Knowledge Exchange: For novice and seasoned hikers, communities become invaluable resources for learning. Tips on gear, trail recommendations, safety protocols, and conservation practices are just a few examples of the knowledge exchanged within these groups.

Conservation and Advocacy: United by a shared passion for the outdoors, hiking communities often become potent voices for environmental conservation, advocating for the protection and responsible enjoyment of natural spaces.

Building a Hiking Community

Creating a hiking community can start with a few individuals and grow to encompass a diverse group of outdoor enthusiasts. Here are strategies to build and sustain an engaging and inclusive community:

Start Locally: Connect with local hikers through social media, local outdoor retailers, or community boards. Organize regular hikes and meetings to foster connections.

Utilize Social Media: Platforms like Facebook, Instagram, and Meetup are excellent tools for reaching out to potential members, organizing events, and sharing information and inspiration.

Inclusivity: Make inclusivity a cornerstone of your community. Strive to welcome hikers of all backgrounds, skill levels, and experiences, ensuring everyone feels valued and supported.

Educational Events: Host workshops and talks on trail safety, first aid, navigation, and Leave No Trace principles. Educating members enhances safety and deepens their connection to hiking and conservation.

Volunteer and Conservation Efforts: Organize group volunteer opportunities with local conservation organizations or trail maintenance projects. Engaging in conservation strengthens the community's bond and commitment to protecting natural spaces.

Nurturing the Community

Maintaining its ethos and supporting its members becomes essential as the community grows. The sustainability of a hiking community relies on continuous engagement, support, and adaptation to its members' needs.

Regular Activities: Maintain an active hikes and social events calendar to keep members engaged. Varying the difficulty and locations of hikes ensure that all members have opportunities to participate.

Mentorship: Encourage experienced hikers to mentor newcomers. This helps novices improve their skills and confidence and reinforces a culture of support and learning within the community.

Online Forums and Discussions: Create online spaces for members to connect, share stories, and seek advice outside of organized hikes. This can help maintain engagement and foster community even when members are not on the trail.

Feedback and Adaptation: Listen to the community's feedback and be open to evolving the group's activities and focus areas. A responsive community can grow and thrive over time.

The Impact of Hiking Communities

The benefits of hiking communities extend far beyond the individual, influencing personal growth, environmental stewardship, and the broader outdoor recreation culture.

Personal Growth: Hiking with a community can challenge individuals to push their boundaries, try new trails, and develop new skills. The group's support and encouragement can inspire confidence and a deeper engagement with hiking as a lifelong pursuit.

Environmental Stewardship: Hiking communities play a crucial role in conservation efforts by fostering a collective respect for the natural world. Members become advocates for the environment, contributing to the protection of the trails and natural areas they love.

Culture of Outdoor Recreation: Hiking communities contribute to a broader culture that values outdoor recreation, health, and environmental stewardship. They can influence public perceptions of hiking, encourage responsible practices, and inspire more people to connect with the natural world.

Building a hiking community is a rewarding endeavor that enriches the hiking experience for individuals and contributes to the collective appreciation and stewardship of natural spaces. Through shared experiences, knowledge exchange, and a commitment to inclusivity and conservation, hiking communities can become vibrant, supportive networks that empower their members and advocate for the responsible enjoyment of the outdoors. As these communities grow and evolve, they carry the spirit of adventure, exploration, and respect for nature at the heart of hiking.

Joining hiking clubs and online communities can significantly enhance the outdoor experience, offering camaraderie, knowledge exchange, and a deeper engagement with the hiking world.

The Benefits of Joining Hiking Communities

Access to Experienced Hikers: One of the primary advantages of joining a hiking club or online community is connecting with experienced hikers. Their knowledge of everything from trail etiquette to gear recommendations can be invaluable for novices and seasoned hikers looking to expand their horizons.

Safety in Numbers: Club-organized group hikes offer an added layer of safety, particularly on challenging or remote trails. There's comfort in knowing that help is at hand should you encounter difficulties, from minor injuries to losing your way.

Structured Learning Opportunities: Many hiking clubs offer structured workshops and training sessions on wilderness first aid, navigation skills, and survival techniques. These learning opportunities are practical and can enhance your confidence on the trail.

Conservation and Advocacy: Hiking clubs often participate in conservation efforts, from trail maintenance to advocacy for public lands. Joining a club can provide a direct avenue for contributing to preserving natural spaces.

Social and Emotional Benefits: Beyond the practical aspects, hiking clubs and online communities offer a sense of belonging. Sharing the trail can lead to lasting friendships, support networks, and an enriching social experience.

Finding the Right Club or Online Community

With the vast array of hiking clubs and online communities available, finding the right fit requires research and self-reflection on your hiking goals and preferences.

Local vs. Global Communities: Consider whether you're looking for a local club that organizes regular hikes in your area or a global online community that offers a broader perspective on hiking cultures and destinations.

Special Interest Groups: Some clubs focus on specific interests, such as peak bagging, long-distance trekking, or family-friendly hikes. Identifying your interests can help narrow down your options.

Culture and Values: Every community has its own culture and values. Spend time exploring a club's activities and ethos to ensure they align with yours. This could relate to its stance on conservation, inclusivity in its events, or hiking approach.

Try Before You Commit: Many clubs offer trial hikes or allow non-members to participate in events for a small fee. Taking advantage of these opportunities can provide insight into whether a club is the right fit for you.

Maximizing Your Membership

Once you've joined a hiking club or online community, actively engaging and contributing can significantly enhance your experience and the value you derive from your membership.

Participate Regularly: Regular participation in hikes and events improves your hiking skills and fitness and strengthens your connections within the community.

Volunteer: Offering your time and skills, whether as a hike leader, event organizer, or conservation volunteer, can enrich your experience and contribute to the club's success.

Share Knowledge: Whether you're a novice or an experienced hiker, sharing your experiences, insights, and tips can help foster a culture of learning and support within the community.

Be Open to New Experiences: Clubs offer various activities, from night hiking to multi-day backpacking trips. Being open to trying new types of hikes can broaden your skills and deepen your appreciation for the diversity of the hiking experience.

Respect Group Dynamics: Being mindful of group dynamics and etiquette ensures enjoyable experiences for all members. This includes punctuality, adhering to the hike leader's instructions, and considering fellow hikers' abilities and preferences.

The Role of Online Communities

In addition to traditional hiking clubs, online communities offer platforms for hikers to connect, share, and learn from each other. These digital spaces can complement the physical hiking experience, providing a venue for discussion, inspiration, and planning.

Forums and Social Media: Platforms like Reddit's r/hiking, Instagram, and specialized hiking forums offer spaces to share stories, ask questions, and connect with other hikers worldwide.

Planning and Collaboration: Online communities can be invaluable resources for planning hikes. Members share trail reports, weather updates, and gear advice. They also offer opportunities for organizing meet-ups and group hikes.

Inspiration and Motivation: Seeing others' hiking achievements and reading about their adventures can be a powerful source of inspiration and motivation, encouraging you to set new goals and explore unfamiliar trails.

Joining hiking clubs and online communities can profoundly enrich your hiking experience, offering avenues for learning, sharing, and connecting with like-minded individuals. Whether through the camaraderie of group hikes, the exchange of valuable knowledge, or participation in conservation efforts, being part of a community can deepen your connection to hiking and the natural world. As you embark on this journey, remember that your engagement and contributions enhance your experience and strengthen the fabric of the hiking community. By fostering a culture of inclusivity, respect, and shared passion for the outdoors, hiking communities can continue to thrive, inspiring and welcoming generations of hikers to come.

Organizing group hikes and events is a rewarding endeavor that fosters community, encourages physical activity, and promotes a deeper appreciation for the natural world. Successfully coordinating these gatherings, however, requires careful planning, consideration of participants' safety, and adapting to unforeseen challenges.

Initial Planning and Preparation

Define the Purpose and Scope: Establish your hike's purpose. Is it a leisurely nature walk for beginners or a challenging trek for experienced hikers? Defining the event's scope will help tailor the planning process to meet your participants' expectations and needs.

Selecting the Trail: Choose a trail that aligns with the group's experience level and the event's objectives. Consider distance, elevation gain, terrain difficulty, and scenic value. Research the trail conditions, weather forecasts, and any permits or regulations that may affect your hike.

Logistics and Itinerary: A detailed itinerary is your roadmap for the day. It should include start and end times, meeting points, planned breaks, and any cultural or natural highlights participants should anticipate. Don't forget to cover transportation options, parking arrangements, and carpooling opportunities.

Safety Considerations

Risk Assessment: Conduct a thorough risk assessment of the chosen trail and planned activities. Consider potential hazards such as wildlife encounters, river crossings, and challenging weather conditions—plan mitigations for each identified risk.

Emergency Preparedness: Ensure that you and other leaders are equipped with first aid kits, knowledge of basic wilderness first aid, and a means of emergency communication (such as a charged cell phone or satellite messenger). Familiarize yourself with the nearest medical facilities and create an emergency response plan.

Participant Preparedness: This is a crucial part of the planning process. Communicate clearly with participants about the physical demands of the hike and the necessary personal equipment. Please encourage them to assess their physical readiness honestly and to inform you of any medical conditions that could affect their participation.

Group Dynamics and Leadership

Establish Clear Leadership: Assign roles within the organizing team, including a lead guide responsible for navigation and decision-making and a sweep to ensure no one falls behind. Clear leadership helps maintain group cohesion and safety.

Fostering Inclusivity: Strive to make your group hikes welcoming to all, regardless of hiking experience, age, or background. This can involve offering a variety of hikes catering to different skill levels and promoting a culture of respect and encouragement.

Managing Group Size: Limit the group size to a manageable number to minimize environmental impact and ensure everyone's safety and enjoyment. Larger groups may require splitting into smaller sub-groups, each with its leader.

On the Day of the Hike

Pre-Hike Briefing: Begin the hike with a briefing that covers the itinerary, trail etiquette, Leave No Trace principles, and a reminder of the importance of staying together. This is also an opportunity to address any last-minute questions or concerns.

Pacing and Breaks: Set a pace that accommodates the slowest hiker and keeps the group together. Plan regular breaks for rest, hydration, and meals, allowing participants to enjoy the scenery and socialize.

Adapting to Conditions: Be prepared to adapt the plan based on actual trail conditions, weather, or group members' needs. This may involve altering the route, taking additional breaks, or, in extreme cases, turning back to ensure everyone's safety.

Post-Hike Activities and Feedback

Debrief and Socialize: Consider organizing a post-hike gathering, such as a meal or informal debrief session. This allows participants to share their experiences, bond further, and discuss future hikes.

Collect Feedback: Solicit feedback from participants regarding what they enjoyed and what could be improved. This information is invaluable for refining future events and ensuring they meet the community's needs.

Promoting and Sustaining Your Hiking Group

Leverage Social Media and Online Platforms: Use social media, websites, and online forums to promote upcoming hikes, share photos and stories from past events, and engage with your community.

Build Partnerships: Collaborate with local outdoor retailers, conservation organizations, and other community groups. These partnerships can provide resources, increase your group's visibility, and support shared goals, such as environmental stewardship.

Foster a Sense of Community: Encourage participants to become active members of your hiking community, contributing ideas for hikes, volunteering for leadership roles, or participating in conservation efforts.

Organizing group hikes and events is a complex process that requires attention to detail, a commitment to safety, and a passion for bringing people together to enjoy the outdoors. By carefully planning and executing your hikes, considering the needs and safety of all participants, and fostering a welcoming and inclusive community, you can create memorable experiences that encourage a love for hiking and a respect for nature. The efforts invested in organizing these events pay dividends through stronger community bonds, increased environmental awareness, and the personal satisfaction of leading successful outdoor adventures.

Volunteering for trail maintenance and conservation efforts represents a critical and rewarding investment in preserving and enhancing our natural landscapes. As more people seek the solace and beauty of the outdoors, the impact on trails and natural areas has intensified, making the work of volunteers more crucial than ever.

The Importance of Trail Maintenance and Conservation

Preserving Natural Beauty: Your regular maintenance efforts help preserve the natural beauty of trails and wilderness areas, ensuring they remain accessible and enjoyable for future generations. You are not just a participant but a crucial part of the preservation process, empowering you with a sense of responsibility and pride.

Environmental Protection: Your conservation efforts play a vital role in protecting ecosystems from the adverse effects of erosion, invasive species, and human activity, thereby maintaining biodiversity and natural habitats. You are not just a bystander but a significant contributor to protecting our environment.

Safety and Accessibility: Well-maintained trails are safer and more accessible to hikers of all skill levels, reducing the risk of accidents and making the outdoors more inclusive.

Tasks Involved in Trail Maintenance and Conservation

Trail Clearing: This involves removing fallen trees, overgrown vegetation, and other obstacles that can block trails and create hazards for hikers.

Erosion Control: Building and maintaining structures like water bars, check dams, and steps are essential for controlling erosion, preventing trail degradation, and protecting surrounding habitats.

Restoration Projects: These projects may include replanting native vegetation, restoring habitats affected by natural disasters or human activity, and removing invasive species that threaten ecosystem balance.

Litter Removal and Clean-Up: Volunteers collect trash left by visitors, helping to keep natural areas pristine and preventing harm to wildlife.

Signage and Trail Marking: Installing and maintaining clear, informative signage helps hikers navigate trails safely and minimizes off-trail hiking that can damage sensitive areas.

Benefits of Volunteering

Personal Fulfillment: Volunteering offers a sense of accomplishment and pride in preserving natural spaces and ensuring that others can enjoy them.

Community and Connection: Working alongside fellow nature enthusiasts fosters community and connection to others and the natural world.

Learning and Skill Development: Volunteers can learn about local ecosystems, trail building and maintenance techniques, and conservation practices, enhancing their understanding and appreciation of the environment.

Physical and Mental Health Benefits: Engaging in physical labor outdoors can improve physical fitness, and spending time in nature has been shown to reduce stress, improve mood, and enhance overall mental health.

Getting Involved

Research Local Organizations: Many national parks, forests, and conservation areas have volunteer programs. To find opportunities, research organizations in your area, such as the National Park Service, local trail clubs, or environmental nonprofits.

Participate in Volunteer Events: Look for scheduled volunteer days, such as National Public Lands Day or local "trail work days," which offer organized contributing opportunities.

Undergo Training: Some organizations offer volunteer training sessions covering safety protocols, tool use, and specific maintenance techniques. These training opportunities can enhance your effectiveness and safety as a volunteer.

Commit Long-Term: Consider committing to a specific trail or area long-term. Regular, ongoing involvement can be advantageous, allowing for a deeper connection to the place and its preservation.

Best Practices for Volunteering

Follow Guidelines and Instructions: Always adhere to the guidelines provided by the organizing body, including safety instructions, tool use protocols, and specific task directions.

Respect the Environment: While volunteering, be mindful of your environmental impact. Stick to established trails, handle plants and wildlife carefully, and practice Leave-No-Trace principles.

Prepare Appropriately: Wear suitable clothing and footwear for work and weather conditions, and bring necessary items such as water, snacks, gloves, and personal protective equipment.

Advocate and Educate: Beyond volunteering, advocate for conservation efforts and educate others about preserving natural spaces. Share your experiences and the value of volunteering with your community to inspire others to get involved.

Volunteering for trail maintenance and conservation efforts is a profoundly enriching experience that offers benefits beyond physical work. It's an opportunity to give back to the natural world that provides solace, adventure, and beauty to so many. The collective effort of volunteers, including you, ensures that trails and natural areas remain safe, accessible, and preserved for the enjoyment of current and future generations. By getting involved, you become part of a community that plays a pivotal role in the stewardship of our planet's precious outdoor spaces, fostering a culture of conservation and respect for nature that transcends the individual and contributes to the global effort to protect our natural heritage.

Elevating your hiking experience transcends simply increasing the miles trekked or summits conquered; it involves deepening your connection with the natural world, enhancing your physical and mental preparedness, and embracing a culture of conservation and community.

Enhancing Physical Fitness and Skills: Your commitment to enhancing your physical fitness and skills is key to elevating your hiking experience. By focusing on these aspects, you can deepen your connection with the natural world, improve your preparedness, and embrace a culture of conservation and community.

Conditioning for the Trail: Building endurance through cardiovascular exercises such as running, cycling, or swimming can significantly improve your hiking experience. Incorporate strength training focusing on legs, core, and back to comfortably handle challenging terrains and long distances.

Mastering Hiking Techniques: Learn advanced hiking techniques, such as efficient backpack packing, proper hydration and nutrition strategies on the trail, and navigation skills beyond primary GPS usage, including map reading and compass use for backcountry explorations.

Adapting to Different Terrains: To become a versatile hiker and gain experience in various terrains—snow, desert, mountains, and forests. Each environment requires unique skills, from using crampons and ice axes on snowy trails to understanding heat management in desert hikes.

Deepening Your Connection with Nature

Mindful Hiking: Practice mindfulness on the trail by engaging all your senses, appreciating the sounds of nature, the texture of the ground underfoot, and the smells of the forest. This deepens your connection to the environment and enhances the mental health benefits of hiking.

Learning the Natural World: Increase your knowledge of the ecosystems you explore. Understanding the flora, fauna, geology, and history of the areas you hike enriches your experience and fosters a greater appreciation for the natural world.

Night Hiking and Astrophotography: Explore the trails after dark for a completely different experience. Night hiking and astrophotography can reveal the wilderness in new ways, showcasing the beauty of the night sky and nocturnal wildlife.

Expanding Your Adventures

Multi-Day Backpacking Trips: Transition from day hikes to multi-day backpacking trips to immerse yourself fully in the wilderness. Planning and executing a successful backpacking adventure requires additional skills, such as camp setup, meal planning, and water purification.

High-Altitude and Technical Hiking: Challenge yourself with high-altitude hikes or technical terrains that require specialized equipment and skills. This could involve glacier travel, rock scrambling, or challenging weather conditions.

International Hiking Destinations: Broaden your horizons by exploring international hiking destinations. Each country offers unique landscapes and cultural experiences, from the ancient footpaths of Europe to the majestic Himalayas or the rugged trails of Patagonia.

Contributing to Conservation and Community

Volunteer for Trail Maintenance: Give back to the trails by participating in or organizing trail maintenance days. Contributing to conservation efforts ensures the trails remain accessible and preserve natural beauty for future generations.

Join a Hiking Club or Community: Being part of a hiking community can enhance your experience through shared adventures, learning opportunities, and friendships. It's also a platform for exchanging knowledge, advocating for conservation, and organizing group hikes.

Advocate for Public Lands and Environmental Protection: Use your passion for hiking to advocate for protecting public lands, conservation efforts, and responsible outdoor ethics. Environmental advocacy ensures that the places we love to explore are preserved and respected.

Cultivating Safety and Responsibility

Advanced First Aid and Wilderness Medicine: Equip yourself with advanced first aid and wilderness medicine knowledge. Being prepared to handle emergencies in remote settings is crucial for your safety and that of others on the trail.

Responsible Hiking Practices: Embrace and promote Leave No Trace principles and responsible hiking practices, including minimizing your environmental impact, respecting wildlife, and being considerate of other hikers.

Continuous Learning and Adaptation: The outdoor world is ever-changing, and so should your approach to hiking. Stay informed about best practices, emerging conservation issues, and new skills to continuously evolve as a hiker.

Taking your hiking experience to the next level is a journey that encompasses physical preparation, skill enhancement, and a deep commitment to the environment and hiking community. It's about pushing your boundaries while respecting and preserving the natural world. By embracing these principles, your hiking adventures become more than just a pastime; they transform into a powerful means of personal growth, environmental stewardship, and community building. Each step on the trail brings you closer to becoming a better hiker, a conscientious guardian of the wilderness, and an advocate for its protection and appreciation.

Hiking, often considered the gateway to the outdoors, fosters an appreciation for nature and opens the door to various related activities and sports. These pursuits range from leisurely walks in the park to adrenaline-fueled mountain adventures, each offering unique challenges and rewards.

Backpacking and Trekking

Backpacking and trekking take hiking to the next level. They involve multi-day journeys through wilderness areas while carrying all necessary supplies in a backpack. These activities challenge hikers to be self-sufficient, navigating remote trails, setting up campsites, and managing food and water supplies.

Physical and Mental Benefits: Beyond physical endurance, backpacking, and trekking cultivate resilience, problem-solving skills, and a profound connection with nature. **Popular Destinations:** Iconic treks like the Appalachian Trail in the USA, the Camino de Santiago in Spain, and the Annapurna Circuit in Nepal offer unforgettable experiences.

Mountain Climbing and Mountaineering

Mountain climbing and mountaineering are natural progressions for many hikers. They introduce the thrill of ascending peaks and navigating rugged terrains. These sports require technical skills such as rock climbing and ice climbing and specialized equipment like ropes, harnesses, and ice axes.

Skill Development: Mountaineering schools and guided ascents can provide the training necessary to tackle high peaks safely. **Community and Teamwork:** Climbing often involves teamwork, fostering a sense of camaraderie and mutual support among climbers.

Trail Running

Trail running combines the cardiovascular benefits of running with the scenic beauty of hiking trails. It offers a faster-paced nature exploration, requiring agility to navigate varying terrains, from forested paths to mountainous tracks.

Races and Events: The trail running community is vibrant and welcoming, with races ranging from local 5Ks to ultramarathons in remote locations, providing goals for runners of all levels. **Cross-Training:** Many hikers take up trail running to improve their fitness, finding that gaining strength and endurance benefits their hiking pursuits.

Rock Climbing and Bouldering

Rock climbing and bouldering involve ascending rock faces and formations using strength, technique, and problem-solving skills. While closely related to mountaineering, these sports often concentrate on shorter, more technical climbs.

Indoor to Outdoor Transition: Many climbers start at indoor gyms before transitioning to outdoor climbs, where they can apply their skills to natural rock. **Environmental Stewardship:** Climbers play a significant role in conservation efforts, advocating access to climbing areas while promoting responsible practices to minimize impact.

Canyoneering and Caving

Canoeing involves navigating through canyons using various techniques, including hiking, rappelling, swimming, and climbing. Similarly, caving (or spelunking) explores cave systems, offering a unique blend of physical activity and scientific discovery.

Adventure and Exploration: Both activities appeal to those seeking adventure and the chance to explore less-traveled paths and hidden natural wonders. **Safety and Education:** Participation in canyoneering and caving requires proper training and respect for the risks involved, emphasizing the importance of safety equipment and techniques.

Snowshoeing and Winter Sports

Snowshoeing extends the hiking season into winter, allowing enthusiasts to explore snow-covered landscapes. Winter sports like cross-country skiing and ice climbing also offer hikers ways to stay active and engaged with the outdoors during colder months.

Accessibility: Snowshoeing is accessible to hikers of all skill levels, requires minimal equipment, and provides a low-impact way to enjoy winter scenery. **Cross-Training Benefits:** Winter sports can enhance endurance, balance, and strength, benefiting year-round hiking and outdoor activities.

Adventure Racing and Orienteering

Adventure racing combines multiple disciplines, including hiking, running, paddling, and cycling, challenging teams to navigate diverse terrains using maps and compasses. Orienteering, focusing on navigation and speed, is a race where participants navigate unfamiliar landscapes using a map and compass.

Teamwork and Strategy: Both sports emphasize physical fitness, strategic planning, navigation skills, and teamwork. **Family and Community Involvement:** Orienteering events, in particular, are family-friendly and cater to various skill levels, making them a great way to introduce younger members to outdoor sports and navigation.

Building a Community Around Hiking-Related Sports

The growth of hiking-related activities and sports has fostered a vibrant community of outdoor enthusiasts. Clubs, online forums, and social media groups provide platforms for sharing experiences, organizing events, and advocating for environmental conservation. Engaging with this community can enhance your knowledge, expand your social circle, and deepen your appreciation for the natural world.

The hiking-related activities and sports world offers endless opportunities for adventure, personal growth, and community engagement. Whether you're drawn to the solitude of backpacking, the challenge of mountaineering, or the thrill of adventure racing, each activity provides a unique way to connect with nature and explore your physical and mental boundaries. By embracing these pursuits, you enrich your outdoor experience and contribute to the stewardship of the natural environments we cherish. As you explore the vast array of activities connected to hiking, remember that the journey is as important as the destination, and the valid reward lies in the experiences and friendships forged along the way.

You are planning your next adventure, whether a serene hike through the local wilderness, a high-altitude climb, or a multi-day trek across diverse landscapes. It is an exhilarating process that combines dreams with detailed preparation.

Setting the Stage: Goals and Inspiration

Define Your Adventure: Start by outlining what you want to achieve. Is it conquering a specific trail, immersing yourself in a new culture, or testing your limits in unfamiliar terrain? Your goal will dictate the nature of your planning.

Seek Inspiration: Look to books, documentaries, blogs, and social media for inspiration. Stories from seasoned adventurers can provide valuable insights and inspire your itinerary.

Logistics: Mapping the Journey

Researching Your Destination: Delve into the specifics of your destination. Understand the best times to visit, the climate, necessary permits, and local regulations. Consider your adventure's physical and technical demands to ensure they match your skill level.

Itinerary Planning: Craft a detailed itinerary, including starting points, daily distances, anticipated challenges, and points of interest. Allow flexibility for unexpected events or opportunities that arise.

Accommodation and Transportation: Book accommodations and transportation well in advance, especially if your adventure takes you to remote or highly sought-after destinations. Consider the logistics of getting to and from trailheads or remote areas.

Training and Conditioning

Physical Preparation: Tailor your training regimen to the demands of your adventure. Focus on cardiovascular fitness, strength training, and endurance. Incorporate relevant skills training for specific activities like climbing or paddling.

Mental Preparation: Mental resilience is as crucial as physical fitness. Practice mindfulness, stress management techniques, and scenario planning to prepare for the challenges and isolation you may encounter.

Gear and Equipment

Essential Gear: Compile a list of essential gear tailored to your adventure. This includes appropriate clothing, navigation tools, shelter, and cooking equipment. Prioritize quality and suitability for the conditions you'll face.

Packing Smart: Balance the need to be prepared with the need to minimize weight. Test your gear before departure, ensuring everything is functional and familiar.

Safety and Risk Management

Understanding the Risks: Assess the potential risks associated with your adventure, including environmental hazards, wildlife encounters, and physical challenges—plan mitigations for each identified risk.

Emergency Preparedness: Equip yourself with a first aid kit, emergency shelter, and communication devices such as a satellite phone or personal locator beacon. Familiarize yourself with the emergency services and protocols in the area you'll be exploring.

Leave a Trip Plan: Always inform someone reliable about your trip plan, including your itinerary, expected return time, and emergency contacts. This step is vital for search and rescue efforts should something go awry.

Environmental Stewardship and Ethics

Leave No Trace: Familiarize yourself with and practice Leave No Trace principles to minimize environmental impact. This includes packing all waste, respecting wildlife, and staying on designated trails.

Cultural Sensitivity: When your adventure takes you through areas with cultural significance or local communities, approach with respect and sensitivity. Learn about the local customs and norms to ensure your presence is respectful and welcomed.

Logistics Revisited: Final Checks and Balances

Review and Revise: As your adventure nears, revisit your plans and preparations. Check for any changes in conditions or regulations at your destination. Ensure your gear is packed and in good condition, and confirm all bookings.

Budgeting: Ensure your financial plans cover all adventure aspects, including unexpected expenses. Having a financial cushion can alleviate stress and provide flexibility during your trip.

Engaging with the Community

Sharing and Learning: Engage with online forums, social media groups, or local clubs in the planning stages and after your adventure. These communities can offer invaluable advice and provide a platform to share your experiences and insights post-adventure.

Post-Adventure Reflection and Growth

Reflect on the Experience: Take time after your adventure to reflect on what you learned about the world and yourself. Consider what went well, your challenges, and how you might approach things differently.

Share Your Story: Consider sharing your story through blogs, social media, or community talks. Your experiences can inspire and inform others, contributing to a more prosperous, connected adventurer community.

Planning your next adventure involves anticipation, preparation, and learning. By approaching your adventure with thorough planning, a commitment to safety, and a deep respect for the environment and cultures you encounter, you can ensure that your experiences are personally enriching but also sustainable and responsible. Adventures have the power to challenge and change us, offering unparalleled opportunities for growth, discovery, and connection with the natural world. Embrace the planning process as an integral part of the adventure, a step that sets the foundation for a truly transformative experience.

The hiking journey is an endless exploration of the vast and varied landscapes that grace our planet and the inner landscapes that define us and who we aspire to become. As we stand at the threshold of concluding this narrative, it's crucial to acknowledge that the true essence of hiking transcends the physical act of walking through nature. It's a transformative journey that challenges, nurtures, and ultimately changes us.

Reflecting on the Power of Hiking

Hiking is more than an activity; it's a gateway to self-discovery and personal growth. Each step taken on a trail is a step towards understanding our capabilities, limits, and the resilience within us. The mountains, forests, deserts, and streams we traverse are not just physical entities; they are teachers, challenging us with their terrains, comforting us with their beauty, and inspiring us with their grandeur.

Through hiking, we learn the art of perseverance. Steep ascents and treacherous paths teach us that challenges, both on the trail and in life, are surmountable with determination and effort. The solitude of the wilderness allows us to confront our thoughts and fears, leading to a profound sense of self-awareness and clarity. The simplicity of being in nature strips away the complexities of modern life, reminding us of what truly matters. Each challenge conquered on the trail is a testament to our strength and resilience, leaving us with a sense of empowerment and accomplishment.

Moreover, hiking is a journey of connection—to the natural world, fellow hikers, and communities that dwell on the edges of the wild. It fosters a deep sense of stewardship for our planet, urging us to protect and preserve the beauty and diversity of our natural environments. Through shared experiences and stories, hiking builds a community of like-minded individuals who value exploration, conservation, and the sheer joy of being outdoors. This sense of community and shared purpose can make us feel connected and part of something larger than ourselves.

Encouraging Readers to Explore Their Paths

The world's trails are as diverse as the individuals who hike them. Each path offers unique lessons, experiences, and joys. Remember that the most profound adventures are often found off the beaten path as you continue your journey. Dare to explore the iconic trails, renowned wilderness areas, and unassuming paths that lie just beyond your doorstep. Every grand or modest landscape has its beauty and wisdom to impart.

Embrace the diversity of hiking experiences. Solo hikes offer solitude and introspection, while group hikes provide camaraderie and shared joy. Night hikes reveal the wilderness in a new light, and multi-day treks immerse you in the natural world's rhythms. Challenge yourself to experience the full spectrum of hiking adventures, for each brings rewards and insights.

Parting Words of Wisdom and Motivation

As you venture forth on your hiking journey, carry with you these parting words of wisdom:

Embrace Each Step: Every step on the trail is an opportunity for growth. Embrace the challenges, the discomforts, and the unexpected turns. They are all integral parts of the journey.

Respect the Journey: Respect the natural world, your fellow hikers, and the communities that welcome you into their lands. Practice Leave No Trace principles and tread lightly on the earth.

Stay Curious: Let curiosity be your guide. Explore new trails, learn about the ecosystems you traverse, and remain open to the lessons the natural world offers.

Share the Journey: Share your experiences, stories, and love for hiking with others. Your journey can inspire and motivate, creating ripples and encouraging more people to explore and appreciate the outdoors.

The Trail Never Ends: Remember that the hiking journey is never complete. There will always be more trails to explore, more mountains to climb, and more horizons to discover. The end of one adventure is simply the beginning of another.

As this narrative closes, know that your journey continues. The trails await, each with its own story to tell and its lessons to impart. May your steps be guided by curiosity, challenges strengthen your spirit, and your heart be filled with the boundless joy of exploration. The journey continues, and it's yours to create.

Creating practical checklists and templates for your hiking adventures can significantly streamline your planning process and ensure you're well-prepared for whatever the trail throws your way. Below are templates for a gear list and a trip planner designed to help you organize and execute your hikes more efficiently.

GEAR
LIST TEMPLATES

This gear list is intended for a day hike in moderate weather. Modify it according to the length of your hike, the specific weather conditions, and personal needs.

Trip Planner Template 1

Basic Gear:

- Backpack

- Map and compass/GPS

- Headlamp or flashlight (with extra batteries)

- Sun protection (sunglasses, sunscreen, hat)

- First aid kit

- Knife or multi-tool

- Waterproof matches/lighter/emergency fire starter

- Shelter items (emergency space blanket, bivy sack)

Clothing:

- Moisture-wicking base layer (top and bottom)
- Insulating layer (fleece or down jacket)
- Waterproof and windproof jacket (shell)
- Hiking pants or shorts
- Extra socks
- Hat and gloves (weather dependent)
- Sturdy hiking boots or shoes

Food and Water:

- Water bottles or hydration system
- Water filters or purification tablets
- High-energy, easily packable food items (nuts, bars, jerky, sandwiches)
- Extra day's supply of food

Navigation:

- Trail map
- Compass
- GPS device (optional)
- Trail descriptions and guides

Extras:

- Camera

- Notebook and pen

- Binoculars

- Trekking poles

- Insect repellent

- Bear spray (if applicable)

- Trash bag (Leave No Trace)

Trip Planner Template 2

Destination Details:

- Trail Name:

- Location:

- Distance:

- Elevation Gain:

- Difficulty Level:

- Estimated Duration:

Date and Time:

- Departure Date:

- Return Date:

- Start Time:

- Expected Finish Time:

Transportation:

- Mode of Transport:

- Meeting Point:

- Departure Time from Meeting Point:

- Parking Information:

Weather Forecast:

- Temperature:

- Chance of Precipitation:

- Wind Speed:

- Special Weather Alerts:

Permits and Regulations:

- Required Permits:

- Permit Obtaining Process:

- Trail Regulations:

Safety Plan:

- Emergency Contacts:

- Nearest Hospital/Health Facility:

- Evacuation Routes (if available):

- Communication Plan (if out of cell service area):

Group Details (if applicable):

- Number of Participants:

- Names and Contact Information:

- Special Needs/Considerations:

Packing List:

- (Refer to the Gear List Template)

Pre-Trip Checklist:

- Inform someone about your trip plan

- Check and pack all gear from the list

- Confirm the weather forecast the day before departure

- Confirm transportation and meeting details with the group

- Download offline maps and trail guides

- Utilizing these templates ensures you're thoroughly prepared for your hiking trip, allowing you to focus on the adventure rather than worrying about what you might have forgotten. Remember, preparation is critical to a safe and enjoyable outdoor experience.

GLOSSARY

This glossary provides a foundation for understanding the terms and concepts prevalent in hiking and related outdoor activities. Whether you're a seasoned hiker or new to the trails, familiarizing yourself with this terminology can enhance your outdoor adventures and conversations within the hiking community.

- **Alpine Zone:** The area above the treeline on a mountain, characterized by harsh weather conditions and sparse vegetation.

- **Approach Shoes:** Footwear designed for hikers and climbers to navigate rough terrain to the base of a climb.

- **Backcountry:** Remote, wilderness areas accessible only by foot or non-motorized means, often requiring more self-sufficiency from hikers.

- **Base Layer:** The clothing layer worn directly on the skin, intended to keep you dry by wicking moisture away from the body.

- **Cairn:** A human-made pile or stack of stones often used as trail markers.

- **Cat Hole:** A small hole dug to dispose of human waste, typically at least 200 feet from water sources, trails, and campsites.

- **Day Hike:** A hike intended to be completed within a day without overnight camping.

- **Descent:** The portion of a hike or climb that involves going downhill.

- **Elevation Gain:** The total amount of vertical ascent throughout a hike.

- **Epic:** A term that describes a particularly challenging or adventurous hike or climb, often with unexpected difficulties.

- **False Summit:** A point along the ascent where it appears to be the summit, but upon reaching it, another higher point is revealed.

- **Fording:** Crossing a river or stream where there is no bridge.

- **Gaiters:** Protective coverings are worn over the lower pant legs and shoes to prevent dirt, rocks, and water from entering the shoes.

- **Glissading:** The act of sliding down a steep slope of snow or ice, usually controlled by an ice axe.

- **Highpointing:** The activity of hiking to the highest point of each of the 50 states in the United States or similar challenges in other regions.

- **Hypothermia:** A potentially dangerous condition in which the body loses heat faster than it can produce, causing a dangerously low body temperature.

- **Inclinometer:** A tool used to measure the steepness of a slope, often found on some compasses used for navigation in the backcountry.

- **Jumar:** A climbing device used for ascending on a rope; not commonly used in hiking but may be employed in technical mountaineering.

- **Knife Edge:** A sharp, narrow ridge or trail section that requires careful navigation due to steep drop-offs on either side.

- **Leave No Trace:** A set of principles designed to promote conservation-minded practices for outdoor activities, minimizing human impact on the environment.

- **LNT:** An acronym for Leave No Trace.

- **Microspikes:** Small, lightweight traction devices that can be attached to shoes or boots to increase grip on ice and snow.

- **Multi-Pitch:** A climb that is longer than the length of one rope and requires stopping at a point to re-anchor is not exclusive to hiking but relevant to mountaineering.

- **Navigation is the** process of planning, controlling, and recording one's movement and position outdoors, typically using a map, compass, and GPS.

- **Out-and-Back:** A trail or hike that leads to a specific destination and then returns the hiker to the starting point via the same route.

- **Packing Out:** The practice of carrying out all trash and waste, including food scraps and used toilet paper, to leave the outdoors as clean as or cleaner than it was found.

- **Peak-bagging Is the** hobby of attempting to reach the summits of a collection of peaks, often within a specific geographic region.

- **Quickdraw:** A piece of climbing equipment used to connect a climbing rope to anchor points; relevant in technical climbing and mountaineering.

- **Rappelling is the controlled descent down a rope in rock climbing and mountaineering. In some regions, it is also known as abseiling**.

- **Scree:** Loose, broken rocks found on mountain slopes, making for unstable and challenging hiking conditions.

- **Switchback:** A zigzagging trail up a steep terrain designed to reduce the slope's steepness.

- **Thru-Hike:** Hiking an entire trail or long-distance path from end to end in one continuous journey.

- **Topo Map:** A topographic map that shows terrain relief, elevations, and landscape features, helpful in planning hikes and navigation.

- **Ultralight Backpacking:** A style of backpacking that emphasizes safely carrying the lightest and simplest gear for a given trip.

- **Vista:** A comprehensive and scenic view, often a goal or highlight of a hike.

- **Water Source:** Natural water sources found along trails, such as streams, lakes, or springs, may require treatment before consumption.

- **Waypoint:** A specific point of interest or location, often marked on GPS devices, used for navigation.

- **X-Country Hiking:** Short for cross-country hiking, referring to off-trail or pathless hiking across the country.

- **Yield:** Giving way to other trail users, following specific trail etiquette to ensure safety and harmony.

- **Zero Day:** A day spent not hiking, typically to rest, resupply, or explore an area without the backpack.

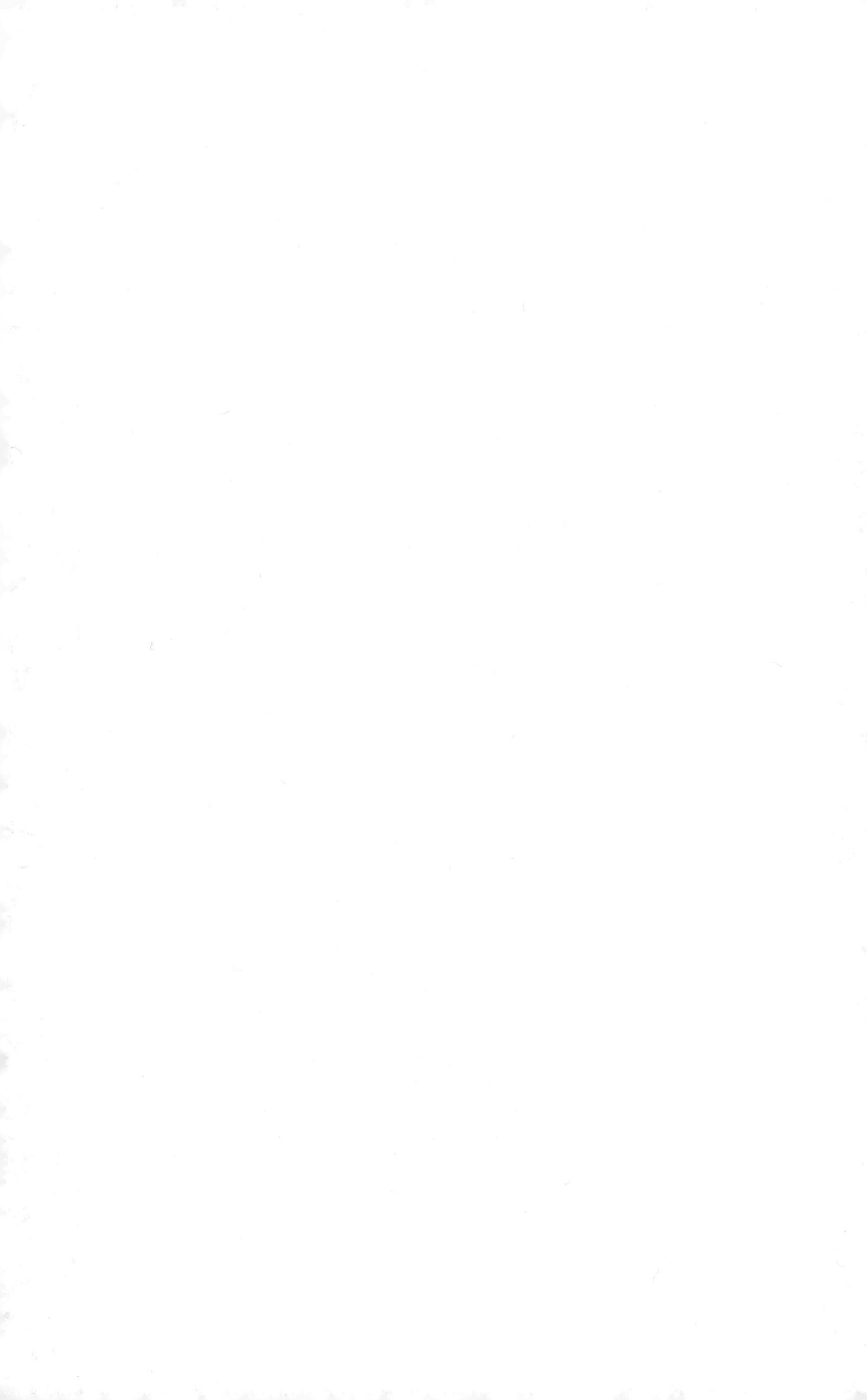